'The way this book is laid out is easy for the reader to understand and follow, allowing the educational and theoretical elements to blend in with the reality of using OT in practice, specifically in music. Throughout the book Jane keeps the language theoretical and factual while still understandable, fun and without waffle. The book also helps us, as students, to understand what is actually important to the individual and gives us stepping stones to start to understand that everything is individual; teaching us to not simply follow a model. I think that this is a captivating and spellbinding book, which contains necessary information and facts along with the added creativity and spark needed to inspire as well as teach.'

– Evie Faulkner, student of Occupational Therapy

'Jane has written this book with OTs in mind, however the breadth of her approach to the whole subject can be appreciated by a very wide audience. The way she explores, explains and brings to life, in accessible language, so many aspects of music means that she has created an invaluable and inspirational resource. For those of us who love music and wish to learn more about its complexities, whatever our perspective, this book will open many doors.'

– Lindsey Stewart, an aspiring singer

'Jane's use of the social model of disability as a means of realising a disabled person's inclusion/participation in music really resonated with me. By the end of this book I wanted to arrange a couple of sessions with Jane myself so convincing was she that music and the environments in which it exists could be adapted in a way that would enable my access to it. As Jane says "everyone who dreams has music"; this book has given me a roadmap to begin my own journey towards realising my own musical dream.'

– Cathy McCormack, deaf occupational therapist, Fulbright Scholar in deaf studies and Gallaudet University graduate

of related interest

Active Support
Enabling and Empowering People with Intellectual Disabilities
Jim Mansell and Julie Beadle-Brown
ISBN 978 1 84905 111 8
eISBN 978 0 85700 300 3

Activities for Adults with Learning Disabilities
Having Fun, Meeting Needs
Helen Sonnet and Ann Taylor
ISBN 978 1 84310 975 4
eISBN 978 1 84642 962 0

Caring for the Physical and Mental Health of People with Learning Disabilities
David Perry, Lousie Hammond, Geoff Marston, Sherryl Gaskell and James Eva
Foreword by Dr Anthony Kearns
ISBN 978 1 84905 131 6
eISBN 978 0 85700 225 9

Exploring Experiences of Advocacy by People with Learning Disabilities
Testimonies of Resistance
Edited by Duncan Mitchell, Rannveig Traustadottir, Rohhss Chapman, Louise Townson, Nigel Ingham and Sue Ledger
ISBN 978 1 84310 359 2
eISBN 978 1 84642 511 0

Promoting Social Interaction for Individuals with Communicative Impairments
Making Contact
Edited by M. Suzanne Zeedyk
ISBN 978 1 84310 539 8
eISBN 978 1 84642 783 1

MUSIC
AND THE
SOCIAL
MODEL

An Occupational Therapist's
Approach to Music with
People Labelled as Having
Learning Disabilities

JANE Q. WILLIAMS

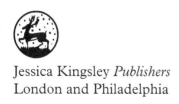

Jessica Kingsley *Publishers*
London and Philadelphia

First published in 2013
by Jessica Kingsley Publishers
116 Pentonville Road
London N1 9JB, UK
and
400 Market Street, Suite 400
Philadelphia, PA 19106, USA

www.jkp.com

Copyright © Jane Q. Williams 2013

Library of Congress Cataloging in Publication Data
Williams, Jane Q.
  Music and the social model : an occupational therapist's
approach to music with people labelled as
having learning disabilities / Jane Q. Williams.
      pages ; cm
  Includes bibliographical references and index.
  ISBN 978-1-84905-306-8 (alk. paper)
  1. Music therapy. 2. Learning disabled--Education. 3. Music--Social aspects. I. Title.
  ML3920.W545 2013
  615.8'5154--dc23
                        2013004564

British Library Cataloguing in Publication Data
A CIP catalogue record for this book is available from the British Library

ISBN 978 1 84905 306 8
eISBN 978 0 85700 636 3

Printed and bound in Great Britain

For everyone who touches my life with their music.

Contents

Preface

Music was an important part of my childhood. At primary school I was, musically at least, a joiner – recorder group, guitar club, choir, orchestra, you name it, I was there. In my teens the cost of music lessons was prohibitive and my musical life focused around my big sister's record player.

I trained as an Occupational Therapist (OT) straight from school and later completed my OT Masters degree. The majority of my 20 years in practice was Local Authority based; an OT practitioner, a supervisor and manager of OTs and Social Workers and finally a Learning and Development Manager.

I'd always imagined myself a sax player and when I was presented with one for my 40th birthday, my life changed completely. Within two years I had quit my job, had two music diplomas (one ABSRM performance, one Open University theory) and had set myself up as a freelance music teacher and facilitator of music groups for people with learning difficulties. None of the work I did required me to have the title of State Registered Occupational Therapist and I wondered if I should let my registration lapse.

As my new life unfolded, I was struck by a number of things:

- Many of the people with learning difficulties who came to the music groups were as passionate about music as I was, but their access to it was startlingly different from mine.

- Music is, and always has been, a fundamental activity in all cultures. Occupational Therapy is concerned with human occupation and purposeful activity and yet a literature search on the words 'Music' and 'Activity' produced a short list of books almost all of which were written by Music Therapists. I found nothing written from an OT perspective.

- And finally, if I started from my firm belief that everyone is musically able and applied my OT knowledge to enabling participation in music then what people were capable of achieving was inspiring.

I've worked as a Music Facilitator for six years and learnt a lot of things along the way. I decided it was time to share some ideas, ask some questions, present a few challenges and tell some stories.

The title of this book

The original working title of this book was...

Music and the Social Model: An Occupational Therapist's Approach to Music with People with Learning Difficulties

The use of the label 'people with learning difficulties' reflects the preferred term chosen by People First for the group of people that People First represents.

The publisher was concerned that many people, particularly in the USA, use the term 'learning difficulties' to describe people who have dyslexia, dyspraxia or attention deficit disorder (the equivalent label in the UK is 'people with specific learning difficulties').

The dilemma was how to title the book to ensure that its content could be accurately anticipated by potential readers.

My preferred title was...

Music and the Social Model: An Occupational Therapist's Approach to Music Inspired by People Labelled as Having Learning Disabilities

This title:

- recognises that the people I work with have inspired my approach to music
- acknowledges that an approach enabling participation in music is relevant to anyone and everyone with an interest in music; it is not a 'special' approach for people with impairments.

Rachel Purtell (Chapter 3) felt strongly that the word 'inspired' is an unhelpful one since the reader may think I am signing up to the disabled people as brave/humbling/sympathy-inducing, etc. stereotype; I hope that if you read this book you will see that I am absolutely not and would not. After some debate we agreed on...

Music and the Social Model: An Occupational Therapist's Approach to Music with People Labelled as Having Learning Disabilities

This title is a compromise that I have agreed to in anticipation that it:

- will mean that the appropriate audience pick it up and read it

- makes it clear that 'people who have learning disabilities' is not a term that I am comfortable with or that I use, but it is a label that society (and in the UK that includes the statutory agencies) often applies to the people I work with.

Labels may be an inevitable part of how we communicate; I couldn't find a title for the book that conveyed the meaning I wanted it to convey without including one. Books written by people who work with the group that a Social Model approach (and I) would label 'people with learning difficulties' continue to use the terms 'people with learning disabilities', 'people with intellectual disabilities', even 'people with mental retardation'. Whilst some of these terms may be enshrined in the legislation of various countries, they are value laden and I personally find them disrespectful, even offensive. These labels are an entirely inaccurate description of the people I work with. In an accessible environment they are creative, quick, surprising, stimulating and funny because that is what people are; I have learnt, and continue to learn a huge amount about understanding music, from each of them.

Language *is* important: it is a reflection of social value. I hope that one of the things this book will do is challenge people, particularly therapists, professionals and people in positions of power, to think more carefully about the language they use and the message they are giving by using it.

Introduction

How to use this book

This is a book that explores the relationships between:

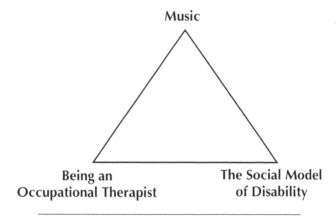

Figure I.1 Music, OT and the Social Model

The most important thing about this book is that you use it. Read it from cover to cover or dip in and out of the bits that look interesting, but please don't just read it. Read it actively, think about what it means to you (feel free to agree and disagree with me wherever you like), take your ideas and use them to make a difference somewhere.

My intention in writing this book was to:

1. Make a difference to how people with learning difficulties experience and access music.

2. Raise the profile of music as a domain of concern for Occupational Therapists.

3. Demonstrate what a Social Model approach to OT practice might look like.

4. Demonstrate the connection between theory and practice from a practitioner's perspective; setting out concepts and ideas and demonstrating

how they can influence and inform practice in a way that can be applied to music or any other activity.

5. Provide ideas about how the complexities of music can be broken down and made accessible.

6. Give examples of music-based activities and music sessions.

7. Illustrate, with stories, some of the things that have worked well.

8. Introduce The LA Buskers.

9. Produce a book that's easy and fun to read.

10. Inspire people to try things out, to have a go and to see for themselves that if you start from the assumption that everything is possible then generally…it is; it's just a question of working out how, and that is what OTs are good at.

What you will find in this book

1. This is a book about *people* and about *music*; it applies the principles of a Social Model approach using the language of people and music. Medical model and deficit model language (e.g. physical dysfunction, functional deficit) will be avoided.

2. The people in the book are referred to by name, as 'people', as 'the group' or as 'the band' as appropriate. They are not referred to as 'patients' or 'clients'.

3. The names used are real. Pseudonyms or references to individual people by letters of the alphabet (e.g. Client X) are not used. It's important to me that people can identify themselves and their stories in this book. The LA Buskers, in particular, are proud of what they have achieved and would like you to know who they are. Some of the stories I've used to illustrate points relate to people I am no longer in touch with. I considered leaving these stories out, but that seemed disrespectful; this book is about what I have learnt through working with them. These people are unnamed in the text because they have not been directly involved in writing this book.

4. Whilst there is a chapter (Chapter 5) that outlines the 'models' that inform my thinking, the processes and approaches described in the subsequent chapters are not framed in the language of particular theoretical models. When it comes to application, the models are used like cookery; an idea here, a bit from there, I wonder if it would be useful to try…etc. I do remember well how often, as an OT student, I was advised against the 'eclectic' approach. This is a book written by a practitioner, not an

academic. Models are applied pragmatically not dogmatically, and whilst this is doubtless an approach that is open to challenge regarding its lack of scientific rigour, I'd defend and actively recommend it on two accounts:

- Part of what we bring to any interaction is our own humanity and part of the richness of our humanity is that we'll always do it our own way.

- Any experience shared at a specific point in time is a one-off event that every person who was there will have experienced differently; experience cannot be standardised.

I'm sure that you cannot objectively measure human experience and I doubt that there is any benefit in doing so in the domain of Occupational Therapy. However, there is a value in being able to track your thinking back to the models that it's rooted in; to be able to give words to ideas so that you can both discuss them with others, and challenge your own way of working by viewing your approach through the range of lenses that different models provide.

5. The writing style is conversational rather than academic. I firmly believe you lose nothing and gain a great deal by describing your ideas in a way that increases the chances they'll be understood. This book is about communicating ideas. I see nothing for any group, professional or otherwise, to gain by developing its own exclusive language. The use of everyday language seems particularly pertinent when describing an OT approach since the profession seeks to be person-centred.

Notes from the author:

- Before you read another word if you have never read Paul Abberley's article: 'Disabling Ideology in Health and Welfare – The Case of Occupational Therapy' (Abberley 1995), I'd strongly advise you to read it now. In 1995, it fundamentally affected the human being and the Occupational Therapist that I was, and therefore the book that this has become.

- Please ensure that appropriate permission is sought before using music that is under copyright.

PART 1

Theory

CHAPTER 1

What is Music?

An overview of the elements of music

Anyone who dreams has music.

Music has been described as 'sonorous air' (Barenboim 2008, p.5, cites Busoni). The dictionary confirms that 'sonore' means 'sound wave' (Latham 2004). Certainly music's medium of expression is sound but can *any* sound then be described as music?

Musicians and composers have often referred to the critical relationship between sound and silence as an essential element in creating music. Messiaen described music as silences framed by notes. Alban Berg, when asked to speak publicly on the future of music, stood and remained silent. Barenboim (2008) describes the critical importance to musicality of the way that notes decay to join the silence or unfold to emerge from it. John Cage's best known composition is probably 4 minutes and 33 seconds, a 'silent' piece composed with the intention of questioning the definition of 'Music'.

So, is there a set of requirements that must be met in order for people to agree that sound or silence is musical?

There seems to be a level of agreement in the music theory literature about the nature of the organisation of sound in space that is required in order that it can be called music. Music theorists approach the definition of music by breaking it down into component parts.

Components of music

The basic elements of music are rhythm, melody and harmony. These are Tovey's three dimensions of music (Tovey 1944), Latham's basic elements (Latham 2004), and Barenboim's triad (Barenboim 2008).

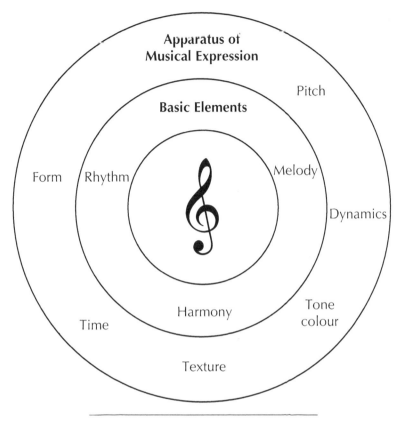

Figure 1.1 The components of music

The basic elements defined

Rhythm: The perceptible organisation of musical events in time (Latham 2004), for example the drums in Queen's We will Rock You or the opening motif of Beethoven's 5th symphony.

Melody: A succession of notes of varying pitch, with an organised and recognisable shape. (Latham 2004). Successful rock and pop songs are sometimes described as having 'a hook' – a repeated melodic phrase (tune) that you can't get out of your head, that you hum as you walk down the street.

Harmony: The simultaneous sounding of notes to produce chords and chord progressions (Latham 2004) (the sound of a strummed guitar, for example).

A second layer of complexity concerns the subtleties in the way in which music is realised. This layer includes pitch, time, dynamics, tone colour, texture. Cooke (1989, p.34) describes these elements as 'the apparatus of musical expression'.

Apparatus of musical expression

Pitch: A basic dimension of sounds, in which they are heard to be high or low (Latham 2004).

Time: Has two aspects: tempo, the speed at which a piece is performed (Latham 2004) and metre (beat), the pattern of regular pulses by which a piece of music is organised (Latham 2004). Metre is the aspect that gets your foot tapping or you can clap along to.

Dynamics: The variation in the volume of the sound (Latham 2004); the rises and falls in volume that build tension. Try listening to a Beethoven symphony on your car stereo without touching the volume control.

Tone colour: (timbre) The quality of sound characteristic of a particular type of instrument or voice (Latham 2004; the solo break in Baker Street has to be alto saxophone).

Texture: The vertical build of music: The relationship between its simultaneous sounding parts (Latham 2004). It's the reason why singing in rounds is so effective and you can't play a symphony on solo kazoo.

Form: The shape or structure of a musical work: The way in which the basic components are organised to make it coherent to a listener (Latham 2004). There are many and diverse musical forms, particularly in classical music. The most familiar form in popular music is strophism where verses alternate with a recurring chorus.

Breaking music down can help to demystify it and make some musical tasks, for example playing a piece in ensemble or writing a song, more easily achievable, yet whole music fulfils the Gestalt principle of being much greater than the sum of its parts. Whilst it's necessary to learn the nuts and bolts to develop basic instrumental skills, becoming an expert performer involves assimilating them into a whole where you understand but are not constrained by the rules. In addition, whilst playing an instrument well is likely to affect the way you listen to or compose music it's not an essential ingredient. Many famous composers and well-regarded music critics are not accomplished musicians. Music has the power to convey emotion; to deliver a message far beyond the technical details. Whilst it may take an expert to deliver the message, human beings seem, often even without basic knowledge of music, to be able to receive it.

It seems to be a rite of passage of every generation to dispute their elders'criteria about what qualifies as music ('they don't make them like they used to', 'the old ones are the best'). New Music (from Stravinsky's The Rites of Spring to the dawning of rock 'n' roll, punk or rap) challenges the accepted definition of what music is by pushing the edges of the rules about how the components of music fit together. New music is perhaps most challenging when it communicates a powerful message. In the western world our right to make new music is linked to our cultural belief that we are entitled to freedom of expression and to have a voice.

The availability of top flight recordings, the pervasiveness of music as background noise and the western addiction to TV talent shows have inevitably influenced what we think music and certainly 'good enough' music sounds like. But...

Has this made us more or less accepting of new and different music?

Has it made us harsh or generous judges of amateur performance?

Has it increased or decreased disabled people's access to music?

Why are there very few well-known bands or classical ensembles that have amongst their number people with learning difficulties? (Heavy Load are exceptional (see Web References)).

Do we, as a society, think that people with learning difficulties are unable to define, learn about or appreciate music?

That they have no interest in it? No message to convey through it?

Are we afraid that their performances will not be 'good enough' to be defined as music?

It would be hard to find a better definition of what music is than to paraphrase Roald Dahl's *Big Friendly Giant* (Dahl 1991) – music is like a langwitch, it is the sound that dreams are making.

Everyone who dreams has music.

CHAPTER 2

Why Music?

The relationship between music and human occupation

In 1990 Professor Elizabeth Yerxa spearheaded the foundation of the new discipline of Occupational Science and presented a 'work in progress' definition of the 'Occupation' in 'Occupational Therapy'. The definition read as follows: 'The specific "chunks" of activity within the ongoing stream of human behaviour which are named in the lexicon of the culture' (Hopkins and Smith 1993, p.49 cite Yerxa *et al.* 1990). The philosopher Aaron BenZe'ev (Hopkins and Smith 1993, p.50) was invited to explore the definition of occupation by answering the question 'what is occupational activity?' His definition was 'a repeated complex pattern of actions whose value is not limited to the value of its external results.' This view presents a challenge for Occupational Therapy, since it calls into question the validity of a focus on DADLs and PADLS (domestic and personal activities of daily living) when they are performed for a purely functional outcome. It also raises the issue of identifying occupations that *do* fulfil the requirements of the definition.

Is music a 'specific "chunk" of activity within the ongoing stream of human behaviour which is named in the lexicon of the culture?'

Is music 'a repeated complex pattern of actions whose value is not limited to the value of its external results?'

Is music 'an occupational activity?…a human occupation?'

In 1977 two un-crewed spacecraft set off to Jupiter. Alongside recordings of greetings in 51 languages the Voyager spacecraft contained recordings of 27 pieces of music. Music was the means by which the human race chose to introduce itself, in all its complexity, to aliens (DeGraffenreid *et al.* 2006). Oliver Sacks (2008) suggests that whilst aliens might wonder why humans occupy so much of their time with music, they could not fail to see that it is central to human life.

References asserting the fundamental importance of music to humanity are not hard to find. DeGraffenreid *et al.* (2006, p.4) suggest that, 'Our ability to create music makes us unique' and 'reflects the very essence of human creativity.' The conductor Esa-Pekka Salonen goes one step further and asserts that music is a biological need. 'It's part of the DNA of our species, because every culture has music. It defines our species as much as the fact we can bend our thumb over our palm – or even more!' (*Amnesty Magazine* 2011, p.38).

Music and human evolution

Making music has been a human occupation for thousands of years. The oldest known musical instruments date back 36,000 years (Mithen 2007). From cave paintings to pyramid murals, man has depicted himself playing musical instruments. Of course we'll never know how the Neanderthals sounded, but Mithen (2007, citing Blacking 1973) is not alone in proposing that the first vocal sounds of early man served the dual purpose of language and song, with song communicating the emotional content of the linguistic message.

Music and society

Darwin (cited by Sacks 2008), ranked human music-making as an evolutionary mystery that served no purpose, in terms of the proliferation of the species and yet was present in every society. Perhaps then music is crucial to the idea of 'society'. A rich inheritance of folk, religious and classical music dating back to medieval times demonstrates that human society was a place for popular music-making long before the arrival of TV talent shows. Across the centuries and the globe, music has been a vehicle for both the ordinary (communicating stories and messages without the need to be literate) and extraordinary (demonstrating wealth and status) business of society.

Music and culture

Many genres of music are so strongly associated with a national identity that just a few bars of music evoke a mental picture of the source culture (consider for example, South American pan pipes, Jewish klezmer, Spanish flamenco, Jamaican reggae, African drumming). The end of the nineteenth century saw English composers (Vaughan Williams, Holtz, Stanford) taxed by the lack of a national sound and feverishly collecting folk songs (The Open University 2002a) and the United States tasking Dvořák, with his reputation for composing strongly Czech music, to develop an American national sound, such was the importance of music to nationalism (The Open University 2002b, cites Tibbets).

Cultural identity isn't confined to nationalism. Culture has been defined as 'the set of customs, beliefs, language, arts and institutions of a group of people that are learned and transmitted within that group' (DeGraffenreid *et al.* 2006, p.24). Any group will have its own culture and usually there is music associated with it. Groups often have anthems, for example football songs, protest chants, school songs, that bring the individuals in the group together in a single voice. Trends in popular music are often so central to a generation that it is the music that is responsible for shaping the language and fashion of that generation; consider rap, glam rock, mods, punk, rock 'n' roll and the Charleston. Music, sometimes, gives rise to a culture.

Music as part of our everyday existence

These days everyone can get their own original works into a public space in minutes, courtesy of the internet. Ease of recording and transmitting music has led to the western world being full of music all day, every day. Sometimes it's unwelcome, arguably it is so ever-present that the ability to listen to it intelligently is being lost (Barenboim 2008). Perhaps this is true, but it is a view that assumes that the primary purpose of *all* music is to be listened to intelligently; some music is disposable. Music can influence without being the focus of attention. It serves many purposes:

- Background noise and to create an atmosphere (in restaurants, shops, hotel lobbies, theatres before curtain up).

- Distraction (call centre queuing music, doctors' waiting rooms, and dentists' surgeries).

- Company (in the car, in the house, on the MP3 player).

- Identity (a personal record collection).

- To create a memorable image (TV advertising: Dvořák's New World Symphony largo has become synonymous with a certain loaf of bread, and J.S. Bach's Air on a G string with a particular brand of cigar).

- To build tension, particularly in films. Consider the music for *Jaws* or the shower scene in *Psycho*.

- To help communicate an emotion (Also Spracht Zarathustra in *2001: A Space Odessy*).

- To tell a story (*Peter and the Wolf*).

- The focus of passive or active entertainment (live bands in a pub, an evening at an orchestral performance, karaoke, nightclubs, discos, barn dances).

- An essential ingredient of any celebration from birthdays to carnivals, Christmas to Hogmannay.

- A focus for worship (e.g. religious music – in any religion from Buddhism to Christianity).

- Part of a ceremony or rite of passage (e.g. weddings, Barmitsvas and funerals).

- A fanfare to announce an arrival (trumpets to announce royal arrivals, church bells opening the Olympics).

- A display of national pride (Shostakovich's 5th Symphony, Elgar's Pomp and Circumstance marches).

- A propaganda tool (Hitler's use of Wagner and banning of Mendelssohn).

This pervasive presence of music in our lives at every key moment is surely evidence of its power.

As with any art form, it is possible to establish connections between the development of music in relation to social, political and technological changes through time, but more than this, music can be seen as a mirror, a reflection of life, 'an expression of the world' (Barenboim 2008, p.5 cites Schopenhauer). On an individual scale, involvement in music-focused activity can support the development of understanding, skills and knowledge that are useful in the world. The transferrable social, physical, emotional and cognitive benefits, whether they are incidental or intentional, can be significant.

Music and memory

Music and memory have a multi-faceted relationship. Significant personal memories are often linked to particular songs – the music can evoke the memory or vice-versa. Music is a useful tool when memorising and rote learning (for example the ABC song). Memory for music often persists in people with dementia long after other memories have lapsed (Sacks 2008).

Music and language

Musicians often learn complex musical rhythms by ascribing words to them (famously, the rhythm of the finale in Beethoven's Violin Concerto is 'it must be jelly, it must be jelly coz strawberry jam don't wobble like that'). There is a demonstrable relationship between musical rhythm and the language rhythm of the culture that creates it (Patel and Daniele 2003). It's difficult, for example, for western Europeans to learn Samba rhythms, because native speech patterns aren't reflected in the rhythms of the music.

Research suggests that babies lose their responsiveness to phonemes that are not part of their native language in their first 12 months (Pallier, Christophe and Mehler 1997), and experts support the view (Goddard-Blythe 2012) that singing to babies stimulates their language development. The relationship may not yet be fully understood but music and language would appear to be intrinsically linked. People who, for whatever reason, cannot speak fluently can sometimes sing fluently.

Music, mood and emotion

It was obvious to the Big Friendly Giant (Dahl 1991, p.107) that 'sometimes human beans is very overcome when they is hearing wondrous music...the music is saying something to them. It is sending a message. I do not think the human beans is knowing what that message is, but they is loving it just the same.'

Music illicits a physiological emotional response that includes an increase in serotonin release (see Web References, Buzzle). Sometimes the human response is a collective one (e.g. the buzz from big feel-good rock anthems or The Last Night of the Proms) as if the music has somehow tapped into some primitive emotional mechanism. Sometimes the reaction is much more personal and might be linked consciously or subconsciously, to a particular memory.

Music can be used as a way of expressing feelings and as a cathartic outlet (e.g. venting frustration on a drum kit, singing out loud at a rock concert, playing the car stereo on full volume on the way home from work). Music can sometimes help personal identification of a feeling (e.g. hearing a piece of music that is relevant at a particular moment). Music also has the power to change mood: to energise or relax, to elevate or calm (Roberts 2004). The serotonin release and rapid, if short-term, lift in mood associated with dancing or singing, is a tonic that pharmaceutical companies find hard to emulate. Music is a means of reaching a peaceful stillness. From Tibetan and native American meditative chants to the western minimal, classical music can be found with the tempo and timbre to relax.

Music and learning

In 1997 publication of a book entitled *The Mozart Effect* (Campbell 1997) spawned a rash of books and recordings in reaction to the notion that listening to Mozart increased IQ. Whilst research has failed to conclusively support or dismiss this claim (see Web References, *The Mozart Effect*), there does seem to be evidence that listening to music stimulates the brain and puts it into a ready-state for learning. Alpha-state Music (recorded at 60 beats/min) is claimed by some (Roberts 2004) to be the ideal music to accompany study. Music is used, particularly with small children, to support rote learning and memorising.

Music and developing an understanding of time

It's no coincidence that people's most relaxed playing tempo matches that of a resting heart beat or that small children can sway in time to music. If time is understood as the rhythm of an unfolding day and night, a week or a season, rather than reading the hands on the clock, then it is inherently linked to music.

Music and developing literacy and numeracy skills

Music can be a useful tool for developing skills in literacy and numeracy. Number songs can be a useful way of illustrating small numbers and simple addition and subtraction (Ten Green Bottles) or of using number as a metaphor for scale (500 Miles, 50 Ways to Leave Your Lover). Melody can add fluency to reading.

Music and the development and maintenance of movement

Music seems to illicit movement in the young, prompting babies and toddlers to spontaneously clap and rock to the beat. Small children are encouraged to develop their skills in co-ordinated movement through the repetition of action rhymes. Music can significantly improve the fluency of movement of people with neurological impairments (Sacks 2008). Learning to play any instrument well involves the development of physical and co-ordination skills.

- Is music 'a specific "chunk" of activity within the ongoing stream of human behaviour which is named in the lexicon of the culture'?
- Is music 'a repeated complex pattern of actions whose value is not limited to the value of its external results'?
- Is music an occupational activity?
- Is music a human occupation?

The answer to all of these questions is surely 'Yes' and if the answer to all of these questions is 'Yes' then the effect of denying access to music would be to disable.

CHAPTER 3

Music and The Social Model of Disability

Rachel Purtell

This chapter explores the Social Model of Disability in the context of access to music by disabled people. The Social Model of Disability is explained, and examples are given to demonstrate its use as a lens through which some of the issues that disabled people face can be viewed.

Traditionally, disability has been seen as the reduced ability of an individual to function and undertake day-to-day social roles when compared to social norms (Oliver 1990, 1992, 2009). The Social Model of Disability focuses instead on the barriers, discrimination and oppression that face disabled people. By thinking about these things, it moves away from ideas about changing or 'fixing' an individual. In this model, an individual's reduced ability to function, their label or diagnosis, is their 'impairment'. 'Impairment' is the word used to define the thing that is about a person's body and/or brain and it always belongs to the individual. 'Disability' refers to the barriers and discrimination faced by 'impaired' people. 'Disability' is something that society can change for the better by, for example, better physical access, people understanding how to communicate with someone who doesn't have speech, or access to welfare benefits.

There is no universal agreement regarding the language used about disability. Sometimes people can feel they have made mistakes or that they have to use specific words without being given a reason. In the Social Model of Disability, 'disability' comes to mean something very specific: it is the impact of society on 'impaired' people. Therefore, the preferred Social Model term is 'disabled people', as opposed to 'people with disabilities'. This reflects the view that disabled people are people who are 'disabled' by the society they live in and by the impact of society's structures and attitudes. People with learning difficulties are 'disabled people' whose impairment is their learning difficulty: they are disabled by the social reactions to it. This view changes the ownership of the problems disabled people face. Disabled people no longer solely own the problems they encounter; they are owned by society as a whole, and society can act to address them.

One of the myths about the Social Model of Disability is that it 'rejects' medicine or treatment: it does not and never has (Oliver 2004, 2009); it provides a lens through which to view all issues that relate to disabled people including medicine. Disabled people are not automatically 'ill' as a result of an impairment. The difference in the way disabled people function as a result of their impairment generally isn't something that is treated or treatable; impairment is not illness. The way a disabled person is will be '*normal*' for them; it is who they are. There is after all no legal definition of 'normal'. The main criticisms of the Disability Discrimination Act (DDA) 1995 (see Web References) were that the definitions of who was covered by the Act were based on diagnosis or function (Marsh 2011) and that it described normal day-to-day activities, but did not define normal. Notions of getting 'better' relate to concepts of a social average function, which is unreasonable and unnecessary (Barnes and Mercer 1996). Disabled people may simply function in a different way and this can lead to social exclusion.

Disabled people, like anyone else, have times of illness and may need to access medical intervention. Ruth Bailey (2012) (see Web References) looked at the issues of clinical access in the NHS and found 'procedures and practices are designed for patients who are ill but non-disabled'. In 'Death by indifference; 74 deaths and counting: a progress report 5 years on' (2012), MENCAP (see Web References) found that the number of people with learning difficulties dying in NHS care due to 'healthcare inequalities' was increasing. There was evidence that people with learning difficulties fail to have symptoms of illness diagnosed because medical staff assume that all their behaviour is linked to their learning difficulties label, or 'shadowing diagnosis' (DRC 2006). Access to basic screening, such as blood tests and blood pressure checks, is sometimes not given. Someone who has no speech and who might not understand a sight test could go undiagnosed and untreated if they develop cataracts, as access to eye tests can be difficult (DRC 2006).

Legislation provides an insight into how society regards disabled people. In *Jepson* v. *The Chief Constable of West Mercia Police Constabulary* (2003) the Police were accused of failing to prosecute doctors who undertook the late termination of a foetus with a cleft lip and palate (Savill 2003). The case centred around The Abortion Act 1967 (see Web References) which set a limit for terminations of a foetus at 24 weeks gestation, unless there is a risk of serious handicap. In England a cleft lip and palate is treatable. The case was lost because the two doctors had acted in good faith when agreeing to the termination, since they believed that the conditions constituted a serious handicap. This poses questions about what level of handicap could be reasonably seen as serious. Scans of foetuses carried out routinely in antenatal care may provide information that could result in a decision to terminate the pregnancy. The implication could be that any abnormality might be considered serious enough to terminate a pregnancy. It is difficult to see how this could have a positive influence on society as a whole. In *Disabled People and the Right to Life*, Clements and Read (2008) describe the 2006 Royal College of Obstetricians and Gynaecologists debate concerning the introduction of active euthanasia for some disabled infants. The Royal College felt the debate was justified because of the emotional burden and financial hardship experienced by families bringing up disabled children. The *Sun* newspaper followed this event by inviting their readers to 'Have your say: do you think disabled babies should be killed?' Clements and Read comment that it is difficult to imagine such a question could be asked about any other group in society.

The Social Model is sometimes criticised for the politicisation of disability and disabled people (Thomas 2004). The model is political and has its origins in Marx's concept of materialism (Barnes and Mercer 1996; Slorach 2011 (see Web References)); disabled people are largely excluded from the means of production, and the evidence for this is that disabled people are likely to be poor and marginalised. Society could change this, but may not act. What gets paid for in terms of care or support systems, what is deemed as cost effective and which needs are considered when making those calculations, and which therapies or treatments are available are ultimately all political decisions. These decisions govern the lives of disabled people. Disability is a political issue.

Luke Clements (Clements 2012) considers that, whilst undoubtedly things have improved for disabled people over the years as a result of developments in service provision and increased awareness of access needs, there are still anomalies in the approach taken by Local Authorities to the identification of need and the provision of support and services to individuals. Clements contrasts a ruling that prisoners should have access to toilets as needed, and not be forced to 'slop out', with another ruling upholding a Local Authority's decision not to provide assistance to a woman to access her own toilet during the night. The Authority provided incontinence pads instead, effectively forcing the woman to behave as if she were incontinent. The justification was that the Authority was entitled to take relative cost into account in deciding whether and how to meet the woman's needs. This raises the question about why any individual's dignity should be accorded less value than that of others.

The theoretical basis of the Social Model primarily comes from people's experience. In 'A Critical Condition' (Hunt 1966), Paul Hunt articulated the injustices and vulnerability (Campbell and Oliver 1996) he had witnessed whilst he was a resident at Le Court Cheshire Home. He questioned why impairment should be the defining factor in what experiences people have and what opportunities are open to them. This question, and the experience of the residents, became the foundation of the Social Model. Hunt, together with Vic Finkelstein and others, went on to form the first Centre for Independent Living. The Centre later became fundamental to the development of what is now Direct Payments for Social Care.

Vic Finkelstein (2001) (see Web References) outlined the concept of the compensatory approach. This is based on the idea that disabled people are 'in deficit' and their situation can be improved by compensating for their personal loss. Examples of this approach in the British welfare system are state benefits, the provision social care and the blue badges parking concession scheme. A move beyond this compensatory approach could arguably be held back by the lack of constructive or affordable alternatives. Simply making something accessible does nothing to change or challenge the underlying discrimination; compensation can support discrimination and oppression (Equality and Human Rights Commission 2009) and actually make things worse. Providing benefits to support people in the workplace has done little to change the willingness of employers to recruit disabled people. In 2010 approximately two million people who were considered to be disabled were claiming benefits for being out of work (The Poverty Site 2010) (see Web References). Reforming welfare benefits may change the compensation for being without work, but not the reason it happens. If doctors want to debate introducing active euthanasia for disabled infants because they and their families face inevitable financial hardship, the compensation approach could be seen to have failed. Currently the compensatory approach is needed as there is nothing else to replace it; this approach poses difficulties, it can and does compensate disabled people for being in an oppression and discrimination of society (Finkelstein 2001; Zarb 2004).

Inevitably, disabled people's access to music reflects these broader themes of exclusion and compensation. The experiences described below were collected from a group of people with learning difficulties, some of whom also had physical impairments. They all had a particular interest in music and some attended a community music group. They became involved in creating a staff training DVD. Two facilitators posed some questions to the group and opened a discussion. Members of the group talked about their experience of music in the widest sense, and also about the principles in the Social of Model of Disability. They began by talking about language.

Has anyone heard the word 'disability' before?

People had heard this word and thought that it referred to 'wheelchairs' and people 'who can't walk' or 'can't hear' or 'can't speak' and 'use signs'. It was a word which applied to other people. There was no sense of any personal connection to this term, despite the fact that for a few people it was to do with a 'blue badge in the car' which they had and used.

What about the words 'learning difficulty' and 'learning disabilities'?

People didn't know what these terms meant. One person thought someone had once used one of these terms about them. It was striking that, whilst most of the members of the group must have heard themselves directly identified with these terms, they had no concept of what they meant. The language is important because it reflects society's understanding. Perhaps society should not label but, in Britain at least, it is often the means by which support and services are accessed. However, people often don't get to choose the words used about them by others and there was no evidence that anyone in the group identified with these terms.

Music festivals or concert organisers may ask for information about a person's 'disability' (meaning impairment) before offering a gratis or reduced cost 'carer' ticket or viewing platform pass. It might be better if 'need' rather than label or diagnosis was the basis for these decisions: 'I am a wheelchair user' rather than 'I have spinal bifida and use a wheelchair,' or 'I get scared in crowds' rather than 'I have an autism spectrum diagnosis.'

Experience of access and attitudes

Restricted access to public transport and campaigning for better access (DAN 2012) (see Web References) for disabled people are well-documented issues. Three members of this group explained how just getting the bus to come to the community music group meant that they experience bullying in the form of name calling from other passengers. One person said that this was the only time they had heard the term 'learning difficulty' when someone had said it about them on the bus and added that sometimes 'people call me spastic'. Most members of the group said this had also happened to them.

Another person said that they only go to the places where they 'know people will be nice'. 'People just bump into you and don't say sorry...people don't talk to me but they talk to the person I'm with...that makes me feel really bad.' Most members of the group agreed that they preferred to go only to places where people are nice to them, and tended to avoid new places.

Only one member of the group had gone to any mainstream events. Concerts and events may often have a single viewing platform for wheelchair users and frequently restrict support to one 'carer', so a family with a disabled parent or child or a group of friends can't stay together.

Expectations of access and attitudes

Most people went to local music activities, or discos specifically for people with learning difficulties and to performances specifically for disabled people. The main arts centre in the city has a very difficult ramped access. Some people talked about going to a 'big gig' to see a famous artist or band, but seemed to believe that this was such a big thing to do that it was unlikely to ever happen. What appeared possible were events that were local, small scale and designed specifically for them.

People also encountered barriers when buying music, either because of physical access to shops or because they didn't have control of their own funding. It hadn't occurred to one member of the group that they should be able to go and buy a CD for themselves.

Experience of staying up late

One person talked about going to a crowded event at the local arts centre and staying up until 11:30 pm 'but I enjoyed it, I had a beer'. The only time another person went to the pub was with a social group specifically for disabled people. A third person said they stay up until 11:30 pm watching films 'and that is fine for me'. Only one person in the group said they had stayed up into the early hours, namely, 3 am. This person goes out with a sibling of a similar age.

Expectations of staying up late

The group was made up of six adults, ages arranging from late teens to mid-forties. They all had a love of music and only one of them had ever stayed up beyond midnight. People seemed to need to justify staying up, as if it was something they needed permission and a specific reason to do. The Stay Up Late Charity campaigns for the right of people with learning difficulties to have the same experiences in this respect that most people would take for granted. The charity tries to challenge the constraints that come from reliance on formal support arrangements (Stay Up Late 2012) (see Web References).

Experience of playing and performing

Two people in the group had their own instruments but hadn't been given any lessons, music books or support to learn to play. They had not thought of asking for lessons. Some people had been given toy instruments and one person had a guitar without strings.

Expectations of playing and performing

Giving people toy instruments or instruments that are not in working order suggests that there is no expectation that they have the ability to learn to play. It's hard to know why anyone should be expected to learn how to play an instrument without proper teaching, but music lessons don't usually appear on people's support plans.

Disabled people are rarely expected to perform; even venues with good audience access usually do not have stage access. On the rare occasions where disabled people do perform, their achievements may be credited to someone else, for example their support worker or therapist (Abberley 1995).

Most performers, at any level of competence, watch other artists and musicians. Many seek inspiration from the people they admire, but for people with learning difficulties, their expectations may be based on very localised and impairment-specific activities, rather than the full range of activities and experiences that most people take for granted.

Expectations in general

Whilst making the training DVD, each person took a role. One young man was director. Directions such as 'Camera, Action' and 'Cut' had been discussed, rehearsed and used throughout filming. At the end of filming a facilitator asked the director, 'What do you say now?' and the director responded, questioningly, 'Thank you?' In itself the 'Thank you' seems polite and innocuous, but it may illustrate something more worrying. Although the director had spent hours working hard both on the film and his role in directing it, his first response was to be grateful and to assume that this is what was expected of him.

The Social Model of Disability was outlined to the group, to see if it might be useful in dealing with the daily barriers they encounter as individuals. A few days later, one of the group members came in and said, 'I told the football club that they shouldn't say I can't come on my own to watch football.' Understanding and applying the Social Model of Disability can lead to change. The Social Model provides an alternative starting point for understanding how society affects disabled people, and prompts questions about how that should and could be different. Social Model proponents are sometimes criticised for not presenting formulaic methods of application or dictating specific actions. Raising the expectation that disabled people can and should have access to everything is a step on the journey towards a more equal society.

CHAPTER 4

Music and Occupational Therapy

Occupational therapy enables people to achieve health, well being and life satisfaction through participation in occupation.

(COT 2004, see Web References)

Music is an occupation rarely used or written about by OTs. A search on the word music on the British Association of Occupational Therapists website on 13 February 2012 produced five references; two were about working with music theatre, one about music therapy, one about music and Parkinson's disease, and one about music and Alzheimer's.

When setting out the scope of human occupation, OT textbooks (Duncan 2011; Hagedorn 1992) sub-divide it into the areas of self-care, productivity and leisure. These are presented even-handedly. Reference to Maslow's hierarchy of needs would support a first priority focus on self-care. In acute hospital settings where the priority is simply to discharge people promptly, a focus on self-care might be entirely appropriate. However, in this setting perhaps it should be acknowledged that the 'client' is in fact the budget holder for the service and not the individual service-user. When the *sole* focus of OT intervention becomes one of self-care then the profession has lost sight of the definition of 'Occupation' (see Yerxa's definition cited at the beginning of Chapter 2).

The occupational values associated with involvement in music include social and cultural values. These aspects of being human should surely feature as a priority when working with disabled people and people with 'chronic conditions', yet, even here, OTs seem rarely to use music as a medium.

Why not music, as a medium for OT?

Service priorities?

- Even in the support of people with long-term conditions, priority is given to health, wellbeing and activities of daily living; those activities that give life meaning, are not prioritised. The long-term occupational support of disabled people, in its widest sense, is neglected. Unless an individual argues that participation in music is essential to their wellbeing (…and they could…) then it is likely to fall off the end of any list of service priorities.

History?

- The OT profession has, through its history, had different relationships with the arts (Hopkins and Smith 1993). A profession that evolved from the arts and crafts movement at the turn of the twentieth century increasingly turned its back on arts and crafts as a medium for treatment in the 1970s and 1980s, arguably in a bid to establish its credibility as a profession. It's past time the profession owned and valued its history, demonstrated a commitment to enabling art-based productivity and leisure and a move back towards a focus on occupation.

Education and training?

- In the 1980s the rhetoric of working with the 'whole person' and doing 'holistic assessment' was in vogue and yet, whilst the author's training involved pottery, woodwork, printing and creative art and placements were spent running quizzes, playing dominoes and skittles, it never once involved an OT music session. It seems highly unlikely that music as a medium has less to offer than these other activities.

Skill and confidence in music-making?

- Most people know some things about music; most people aren't great musicians or composers.
- Many OTs do have music as a large part of their own human occupation and could be using their experience to improve the access of others to music.
- OTs who aren't musicians may lack skill and confidence in music-making and yet many OTs feel skilled and confident enough to facilitate art, creative writing, gardening and cooking sessions…without thinking themselves an expert (or even simply competent) in the medium.

Rejection of a single-medium approach?

- It's a step further to consider the use of music as a single medium for an OT. Single-medium therapy challenges the assertion that OTs are concerned with the 'whole person'.

- Yet OTs have historically embarked on single-medium endeavours (e.g. light and heavy workshops, remedial games).

- Using an approach and a knowledge base that is about being an OT and using it to enable access to the single medium of music, an ever present cultural and social occupation, is surely relevant to the 'whole person'.

Music therapy?

- The assumption is that if the medium is music, then the activity is Music Therapy. Perhaps OTs have avoided the use of music because of this tension. Disability Studies has accused The Professions Allied to Medicine of needing to claim their own exclusive territory in order to shore up their professional status and confidence (Abberley 1995). There is room for everyone to use music as a medium and an OT working with music will always be an OT.

- Music therapists specialise in music; they are few in number and offer a very specific kind of intervention to a small number of people.

Why music as a medium for OT?

- Music is an important human occupation.

- Participation in music gives people a space in which they can demonstrate their capability. The confidence and skill developed in doing so transfers to other aspects of life.

- People with impairments are significantly disabled in terms of their access to music (see 'Music and the Social Model of Disability', Chapter 3), and this has the cumulative effect of excluding them from other aspects of belonging in a culture. Challenging this kind of discrimination is exactly the business of Occupational Therapy.

- An OT view of music as human occupation will add value to the experience of disabled people, particularly when this OT view comes from a Social Model perspective.

- Music provides a huge resource of material and a vast range of activities.

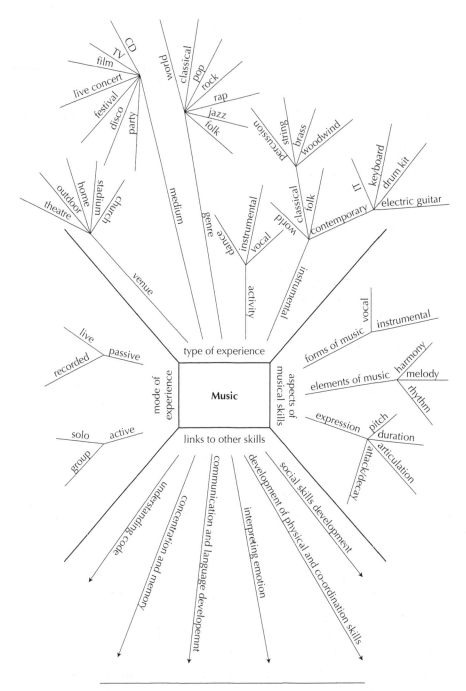

Figure 4.1 Music as a resource for activities

Any aspect can provide the material for activities that can be broken down into manageable steps. Participating in music-based activities can require a broad range and combination of social, physical, emotional, cognitive and musical skills from the simple to the complex.

- Accessible music gives everyone a place where they can succeed.

- Music is a great motivator. Most people react to music. Most people know some songs and have a CD collection. Music is energising.

- Just listening to a performance provides auditory, visual and vestibular (vibrational) stimulation. Playing an instrument adds proprioception, co-ordination and even olfactory stimulation to the mix. Music lends itself to a multi-sensory approach; maximising the range of sensations an activity stimulates increases the likelihood that it will be accessible to a broad range of people.

- Music can easily be used to increase the multi-sensory appeal of other activities, for example exercise or doing the chores.

But perhaps most importantly…

- Music gives people a voice. It gives the 'silent' a means of communicating which not only need not rely on words, but can convey meanings that are beyond words.

And finally music is fun and 'fun is good!' (Seuss 1960, p.51).

CHAPTER 5

The Occupational Therapy Tool Kit

Paradigms, frames of reference and models of practice

This chapter sets out an overview of the shapes, ideas and theories I use when I'm thinking and working. It is not a comprehensive introduction to any theoretical approach; rather it outlines the resources I carry in my tool kit and apply to the work I do and gives references, so these can be read in detail if required.

For the purposes of this book the terms used are defined as follows:

- **Paradigm**. The most fundamental beliefs of the OT profession.

- **Frames of reference**. The theoretical or conceptual lenses through which practice and process are viewed.

- **Models of practice**. The specific occupation-focused constructs and propositions that inform and support practice and process.

Frames of reference and models of practice provide a way a way of seeing the world. Part of what makes a practitioner a professional is the ability to monitor their own approaches, to go back to theory, to challenge their own assumptions and to task themselves to think differently (Schon 1983). Without challenge there is a danger that practice becomes stale, static and inflexible or that the models used become so well-assimilated into a practitioner's thinking that they are no longer articulated and are applied without thought. Having a tool kit of approaches, knowing what's in it, reviewing and updating it and keeping it in good working order is an essential part of practising well.

The paradigm

The most fundamental belief of the OT profession is that humans need to engage in meaningful occupation. The preceding chapters of this book argue that music is a fundamental human occupation.

Frames of reference

The primary lens through which this book views and applies models of practice is the Social Model of Disability. However, there is a valid role for the Medical Model too. Appropriate use of knowledge regarding diagnostic labels can be invaluable in understanding why something happens as it does and being able to present accessible information, ideas and activities (see diagnosis or impairment specific approaches below) thereby increasing the chances of individual achievement. This is perhaps particularly important in the early stages of working with someone; success increases confidence and willingness to experiment.

Models of practice

Models of practice are the ideas and theories that can be used to inform how a task is broken down into achievable chunks or how an activity can support the development of specific skills. Unlike Duncan's 'conceptual models' (Duncan 2011) many of the models described here are not specific to OT. They, like the frames of reference, have developed outside the profession but can be usefully applied. Inevitably, if conceptual ideas are useful they will be widely used by people from a variety of knowledge bases; professional exclusivity seems illogical. Regardless of its origin, a model used by an OT will be applied with the underpinning knowledge of OT.

Types of conceptual model

For ease of reference, the models in the tool kit have been divided into categories. The categories outline the type of models and where they might be usefully applied.

1. **Overarching models**. Give a context to the area of activity and sometimes give a language that can be useful in communicating about it.

2. **Models for prioritising**. Provide a methodical process for working out what to focus on and where to start.

3. **Models for reasoning**. Provide approaches to understanding situations and questioning assumptions about the what, why, how and when.

4. **Models that shape intervention**. Support reasoned approaches to analysing, breaking down and learning skills.

5. **Approaches to learning**. Give information about how to create environments that support individual learning.

6. **Models specific to a diagnosis or impairment**. Inform intervention approaches that are specifically tailored to an individual's impairment or impairments.

1. Overarching models

Conscious use of self

The OT should act as a resource in the interaction between the individual and the environment by contributing their knowledge and ideas of the activity or the process. This knowledge, applied in tandem with the individual's expert knowledge of themselves contributes to the individual gaining maximum value from the experience. In taking this role the OT needs to be acutely aware that their own attitudes and behaviour can shape the experience and also to acknowledge and manage their own needs (To be the expert? To be needed? To be appreciated?) (Hagedorn 1992). Ultimately a good OT will facilitate the independence of the individual and leave themselves redundant.

The model of human occupation (MOHO)

Since the 1980s no OT text would be complete without mentioning MOHO (Kielhofner 1985). MOHO and the academic writing that supported its development took the understanding of occupation and the role of OT to a new level. Whilst the language of MOHO is jargon-laden and inaccessible, the theory of the individual as an open system and the subsystem breakdown into volition, habituation and performance provides a useful framework for building an understanding of an individual's occupational interaction with their environment.

2. Models for prioritising

Meaningful intervention reflects an understanding of the priorities, motivations and aspirations of the individual. The use of shapes for prioritising that are premised on this assumption helps to ensure that this is a value that is applied.

The Canadian Occupational Performance Measure (COPM) provides a process to support an individual prioritisation of importance, a rating of satisfaction with performance and a method of cross-referring the two. This can be used to understand and negotiate individual priorities for intervention. It also provides a useful starting point for checking detail (do you want to learn chords or to play a particular song?) and for weighing up the merits of different interventions (to teach skills or to adapt equipment).

The KAWA River Model cites Social Model references and reflects a Social Model view of disability (Duncan 2011, p.121). The river metaphor is an attempt to develop a model that has cross-cultural relevance. The use of metaphor has its limitations particularly when working with people who are much more able to deal with the concrete than the abstract and who find analogy very difficult to understand (see models specific to working with people with autism spectrum diagnoses). However, the model does use everyday language and avoids professionalising jargon. Its value lies here in its acknowledgement of the Social Model and its use of language; these are important principles for a Social Model approach to OT practice.

Maslow's Hierarchy of Needs and theory of motivation is a useful reminder that it is essential not only to identify individual aspiration, but also to ensure that basic needs are met well enough, so that the individual is free to focus on other things (see Chapter 7, 'Creating an Enabling Environment').

3. Models for reasoning

Reflective practice and clinical reasoning

Clinical reasoning literature (Mattingly and Flemming 1994) gives a language to reasoning approaches. This enables articulation of thoughts and also raises consciousness of how applying a different reasoning approach can lead to the screening in and out of information and the re-framing of presenting situations. Through reflection the practitioner can identify and challenge themselves (Schon 1983). Writing, filming and discussion can help ensure that practice remains creative, open-minded and responsive.

Critical incident analysis

Critical incident analysis was promoted in Health and Social Care in the 1990s as a method for identifying specific learning from inter-agency working. By focusing on an event participants engage in discussion that is based on specific, if subjective, evidence rather than general impressions. The event need not be critical; it's the analysis that's critical. The event can be something that didn't go as well as expected, it can equally be something that went really well or something routine that happens every day. The value of the analysis is in developing a shared understanding of the factors that make things more or less likely to have both a smooth process and a positive outcome.

Models for describing scenarios and processes

Management theory (Mullins 1999) is a useful resource of models for:

- Understanding scenarios (problem identification and analysis).
- Identifying priority action (gap and impact analysis, continuous improvement approaches).
- Measuring outcomes (evaluation approaches).

Like therapeutic models they provide a framework for thinking, for re-framing situations in order to develop understanding and to support the generation of ideas for action.

4. Models that shape intervention

Play behaviour

In 1932 Parten (Hopkins and Smith 1993 cites Parten) proposed a sequence for the development of play behaviour. The sequence begins with unoccupied play, where the individual seems not to play actively but fleetingly observes the activity of others and goes on through onlooker play, solitary play, parallel play and associative play to reach co-operative play. The sequence is a useful one for identifying the developmental level at which the individual is comfortable to operate. Understanding this can help to ensure that activities are presented in an accessible way and that opportunities for the individual to explore less comfortable ways of behaving and interacting are presented in a logical order and are well supported.

Social skills development

The interactive approach (Hagedorn 1992) proposes that the skills required to interact with other people develop through experience. Interacting with other people in a structured group environment is therefore a good way of gaining these skills. Within a group environment positive interaction can be modelled (Bandura, cited by Hagedorn 1992).

Group processes

Berne (1985) wrote extensively about both the development of a group and the roles taken by individuals within the group. The process of forming, storming, norming and performing is a useful one to bear in mind particularly when a group is open and membership changes. The developmental phase of the group can directly impact on the ability of the individuals within the group to focus on an activity.

Within a group setting people take on roles. There are those who like to be centre stage, who observe, who clown around, who will try anything, who challenge, who timekeep, and who look after everyone else. The roles that individuals adopt change, and groups can be a safe and positive place to try out different roles and to feel the effect of different behaviours.

Intensive interaction

Intensive interaction (Caldwell 2008) promotes the importance of observing and understanding an individual's body language and communication. The approach encourages consideration, from the individual's perspective, of both why people communicate as they do and the meaning of the message that they are conveying. It assumes the necessity to be alongside people; doing things and seeking to understand things their way rather than imposing any notion of correct, expected or acceptable behaviour. It defines 'challenging behaviour' only as a challenge in terms of understanding. It is an extremely positive and useful approach when working with people with little conventional verbal language, with people who are labelled as having 'challenging behaviour' and with people who have autism spectrum diagnoses.

The neuro-developmental approach

The neuro-developmental approach (Hagedorn 1992) proposes that the acquisition of physical skills (fine and gross motor skills and co-ordination) follows a developmental sequence. Bobath (Hagedorn 1992) emphasised the importance of crossing the mid-line and of the development of movement occurring proximally to distally (core stability and sitting balance before fine finger activity, for example). Applying neuro-developmental principles informs ideas about how to set up an activity (in terms of positioning of individual and equipment) and how to pitch an activity (by reflecting a developmental stage that is physically achievable).

Sensory integration theory

Sensory integration theory (Ayres 1979) explores the idea that people's experience is enhanced by integrated, multi-sensory stimulation. The integrated use of sound, vibration, movement and visual stimulation can increase confidence in movement, dexterity and vocalising. This theory can inform working with people who experience hyper-sensitivity in both understanding their experience and in planning how to communicate effectively without triggering sensory overload. The use of objects of reference (e.g. giving someone the keys as you say you are going out, a towel to offer a bath, etc.) to give consistent cues about activities, tasks and structure is also useful.

Adaptation and compensation

Adaptation and compensation (Duncan 2011) is an approach that uses techniques including adaption of tasks, cueing, imitation, compensation techniques and adapting the environment (equipment) in order to make activities accessible.

5. Approaches to learning

The behavioural approach assumes that all behaviour is learnt (Hagedorn 1992). It proposes that behaviour can be broken down into a sequence of individual actions and that positive reinforcement of desired behaviour increases the likelihood that they will be repeated. Backward chaining works on the assumption that the positive reinforcement gained from an activity is in its completion. Therefore, if an individual is to get maximum satisfaction out of an activity they undertake with support, the final step to complete it is the most important one for them to do. When planning activities that have several steps, it is important to provide enough support in the early steps of an activity so that the individual has enough energy, enthusiasm and concentration to complete the final step.

Learning styles are much discussed in training, learning and development and management training. Kolb's learning cycle (Kolb 1984) sets out diagrammatically a description of the range of preferences individuals have for how they do things and how they think about things – watching, thinking, experimenting, feeling, and doing. It provides a useful addition to the multi-sensory approach when considering methods for teaching a new skill.

6. Models specific to a diagnosis or impairment

(i) Conductive education

Conductive education evolved in Hungary as a result of criteria for entering state education. In order to get a state school place, children had to walk. The result was an approach where walking was the priority and the personal cost of doing so was irrelevant. It's no surprise then that it's an approach that's slated in the disability studies literature (Oliver in Swain et al. 1993). However, the notion of rhythmic intention not only works in freeing up people's movement, but it is part of the inherent power of music. Sacks (2008, p.270) refers to this phenomenon as 'Kinetic melody': the way in which movement flows and the way in which music can assist this flow, where it is otherwise lacking is sometimes very striking (see Darren's journey, Chapter 9).

(ii) Models, ideas and approaches specific to working with people with autism spectrum diagnoses (Roth 2010)

EXTREME MALE BRAIN

The theory explains some of the characteristics often observed in people with an autism spectrum diagnosis in terms of stereotypical male interests (machines, gadgets, numbers and timetables) and proposes that people with an autism spectrum diagnosis are likely to score very highly on a scale that measures these interests and abilities (systemising) and to gain low scores on a scale that measures features associated with empathising. People with an autism spectrum diagnosis often demonstrate a strong preference for focusing on detail rather than broad concepts.

THEORY OF MIND (TOM)

The approach proposes that people with autism spectrum diagnoses may be unable to second guess the thoughts, beliefs and intentions of others and may assume that everyone has the same thoughts as them. This combination can make social situations difficult or impossible to understand and participate in.

Extreme male brain theory and TOM can help to frame approaches to communicating and presenting both information and activities. They may also yield insight that can inform critical incident analysis.

PICTURE EXCHANGE COMMUNICATION SYSTEM (PECS)

PECS is an intervention technique that maximises the likelihood of effective communication about the structure and content of a day by providing uncluttered pictorial cues. The approach is helpful in conveying information regarding, for example, an activity programme. Used consistently, PECS can greatly reduce the anxiety levels of individuals who otherwise find it difficult to make sense of the structure and unfolding of a day.

The contents of my tool kit are cross-referred in the text of Part 2 (Practice), so that application of the theory to practice is illustrated.

CHAPTER 6

A Social Model OT Process

There is little variation in the representation of the OT process in textbooks (Hagedorn 1992; Hopkins and Smith 1993; Duncan 2011 cites Creek). Fundamentally, it's a generic problem-solving approach for the process of working through what to do (assessment), how to do it (goal planning), doing it (intervention), checking whether it's done (evaluation), calling it done and then moving on (discharge). It can be applied to cooking the tea, getting your hair done, decorating the bathroom – it's an everyday process. Occupation is the substance of our everyday, and in that respect, it seems an entirely appropriate way to frame a conversation between two people about the things that one would welcome the support of the other to achieve. There are, however, a number of issues presented by the medical model interpretation of this process that McCormack and Collins suggest (2010) continue to pervade OT textbooks. OTs who seek to work from a Social Model perspective need to address these issues.

Social Model issues with the OT process

From a Social Model perspective, it's pragmatic to have a process as long as it's not prescriptive and rigidly applied. A declared approach makes it clear to people how the professional sees their role and makes it possible to stop, check and re-position, if necessary, en route, like following a map. The process is sometimes drawn in a linear way (Creek's diagram in Duncan 2011), sometimes cyclical (Hagedorn 1992) but both imply a tidiness and an inevitable, time-limited, journey towards discharge that may be more applicable to acute medical settings and the management of short-term illness or injury, than to working with disabled people.

Roles of individual and professional

Labelling the process an 'OT process' implies that it is owned by the OT. Textbook phrases such as 'the clinical judgement of what is to be assessed' (Duncan 2011, p.37) and focusing on 'identification of the problem' and 'problem formulation' supports that this is the case. Whilst the Creek diagram

(2003) used by the College of Occupational Therapists has a sidebar stating 'implementation in partnership with the client' the idea of 'involving clients' is sparse in the narrative until after an assessment has been undertaken. The 'OT process' label also implies a centrality of that process to an individual's life: it's essential to remember that people's lives are multi-faceted and any OT involvement is likely to be very limited in both the length and breadth of its relevance and impact on a whole life. Perhaps though, OT ownership of the process could be seen as serving a positive Social Model function; it may establish the boundaries of professional involvement, defining the role and viewing the professional as a tool, a means by which an individual can be supported to achieve some of their goals.

Problem orientation and location of problem

Inevitably a problem-solving approach creates a process which is problem-orientated. In Social Model terms this raises two issues:

- The focus on problems without consideration of strengths. OT texts do tend to talk in terms of problem identification. Arguably, even a needs-led approach, when used in tandem with prioritisation and eligibility criteria is likely to focus on problem identification and resolution. OT models that present a more rounded approach, focusing on individual and network assets and resources as well as on issues, remain rare; the KAWA River Model (Duncan 2011) is exceptional in this regard.

- The Social Model is a problem-solving approach, but where the Social Model would view the 'problem' as a societal responsibility the traditional OT/medical approach locates it with the individual. Texts (Duncan 2011, p.5) that present the concept of 'dysfunction' as the opposite of 'competence' (and therefore synonymous with incompetence) represent the polar opposite of a Social Model approach.

Goal planning and evaluation

In order for the achievement of goals to be evaluated they need to be measureable. Traditionally this has meant that goals were behavioural and SMART (Specific, Measurable, Achievable, Relevant, Time-limited). Modern texts (Duncan 2011) are less specific and do refer to the need for goals to be collaborative. Duncan makes a helpful distinction between individual evaluation and service evaluation. If the setting of goals and the subsequent evaluation of their achievement is a service requirement, then openness about this is essential in ensuring that individual evaluation is not compromised. Sometimes service-orientated goals are necessary because:

- Funding depends upon providing evidencing of results.

- The service manager requires it (perhaps to secure funding or as a way of managing staff performance).

- Individual professionals want feedback about the value of their involvement.

- Intervention is contributing to a bigger plan for an individual; a care plan, for example, where a specific intervention may be seen as means of meeting an identified need.

- The individual has a set of things they want to achieve.

- They give the individual and the professional a forum for exploring their work together.

There is a danger though that a simple, behavioural, quantitative approach to service evaluation undermines the value of individual, qualitative experience and consequently fails to inform appropriate Social Model service development. The time limited component of a goal, particularly in rehabilitation services, may result more from service priorities and time scales than from individual needs. A significant number of OT research articles continue to evaluate the effectiveness of intervention by mechanistic measurement (e.g. percentage increase in joint movement); surely no individual measures their occupational performance or their quality of life in these terms. The Canadian Occupational Performance Measure (COPM) (Law *et al.* 1990) provides a positive approach to doing this differently. The individual identifies specific tasks or activities, rates their importance and their degree of satisfaction with performance. This information can be used to both prioritise individual goals and to evaluate the impact of intervention, from the individual's perspective.

Intervention approaches

Intervention approaches are often functional and tend to intervene at the individual rather than the societal level. The KAWA River Model (Duncan 2011) is the OT model that acknowledges disability studies and cites Social Model references which would suggest a move towards a more Social Model approach. However, whilst the assessment approach reflects Social Model thinking, reference to case studies that illustrate the application of the model (see Web References, KAWA Model) tend to focus on the use of KAWA in assessment and problem identification, and intervention approaches seem traditional. Applying a Social Model approach to the OT process but retaining intervention approaches that are medical, rehabilitation or adaptation based may improve the individual's experience of the OT process, but as yet, the profession seems not to have developed Social Model approaches to intervention; this is a significant gap in OT practice.

Language

Inevitably, over time, words become coloured, sometimes tainted, with a particular nuance. The words of the OT process (assessment, goal planning, and perhaps particularly intervention) sound very 'done to'. As Duncan (2011) suggests the chosen use of the word 'intervention' (rather than treatment or therapy) is perhaps the most honest one since, whether it's a welcome one or not, intervention is an intrusion. Perhaps the whole process is an intrusion. The word used to identify the individual has undergone several re-inventions too (patient, client, service-user). The use of 'individual' or 'person' is attractive, but perhaps 'service user' is more appropriate; the individual is part of the process because, whether it's welcome or not, they are accessing a professional service.

Ultimately though, it's the experience of the process that colours the meaning ascribed to the words it uses. In time, experiencing a user-led process would change the nuance of its language. However, the very fact of a 'professions language' will remain divisive. It sets apart, it creates an 'in crowd' (and therefore an 'out crowd'), and it helps perpetuate a power imbalance. The language of a profession that is allied to its community (Finkelstein 1999), rather than to medicine, would use the language of that community; no Babel fish (Adams 1995) required.

Discharge

Perhaps the issue with discharge is also with the meaning ascribed to the word; the professional signing the individual off their books once the problem is solved. It implies that people need to be and can be 'fixed' or, as Paul Abberley (1995) asserted, can't be fixed and have, therefore, failed in some way. The concept of 'signing off' may have its usefulness in an acute environment, where the 'client' is the budget holder/service manager but the connotation of the word, when applied to work with an individual, is one of power imbalance and this needs to be re-dressed if the term is to be useful to disabled people.

A Social Model OT process?

A Social Model OT process would focus on creating a barrier-free environment for all, rather than seeking to cure or care (Finkelstein 1999).

Shape and flexibility of the process

Importantly, the process would not be linear or cyclical. Developments in one area affect others: people's dreams, aspirations, interests, frustrations and opportunities move and change; that's life. To assume that the experience of disabled people is in some way different, to assume they have static needs, frustrations and goals would be to deny their humanity. The process would instead, reflect a life journey. The OT would be involved as and when it was useful and would be represented, accurately, as a minor player, invited in as and when involvement was useful.

Perhaps the process would be better represented like this:

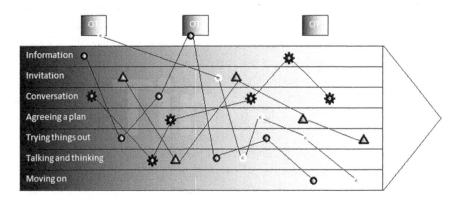

Figure 6.1 Social Model OT Process

Roles of individual and professional

A Social Model OT approach would recognise the individual as the lead. The relationship would not be one of equal partnership; the professional would act as a resource and enabler.

Problem orientation and location of the problem

The approach would focus on assets and see problems as being located in society, not belonging to the individual.

Goal planning

Individual goals and measures of satisfaction (e.g. COPM) may give power to the individual. It could also be argued that goals are important so there is clarity for all involved about direction of travel, but real life isn't always that tidy. Some people are naturally more goal-directed than others; many people just take opportunities as they unfold.

Language

A Social Model OT process would use language that:

1. is empowering
2. is owned by disabled people.

TABLE 6.1 SOCIAL MODEL OT PROCESS

Traditional OT process terms	A Social Model OT process?
Patient, service-user, client	Service-user is the term chosen by the disability movement
Information	Information – about what's on offer and how you can get some of it
Referral	Open access Self-referral Invitation
Assessment	Assessment Conversation Exploration
Goal planning	Agreeing a plan
Intervention	Following the plan Trying things out
Evaluation	Talking about how it's going and thinking and talking about what to do next
Discharge	Moving on

Process and intervention approaches

A Social Model OT referral system would be open-access and supported by good information about what the service might deliver. The system would offer personal invites, taster sessions and drop-in, in order to increase accessibility.

Assessment, conversation, agreeing a plan and trying things out are all parts of an organic, ongoing interaction. Trying things out is particularly important. Poor access to opportunities may mean that disabled people lack the experience to make informed choices about the action they want to take or the things they want to achieve.

Intervention approaches are perhaps the biggest challenge. Intervention within a pure Social Model approach would be at a societal, rather than individual, level and would focus on creating enabling environments through challenging the systems and values of society and seeking legislative and policy change. Perhaps the emergence of the concept of occupational justice within the profession will move this agenda forward. Such an approach to intervention would require a significant change in the way that OT involvement is funded and its effectiveness measured. In the absence of that change, intervention must seek to resolve problems from a starting point of societal rather than individual ownership of them.

Moving on would be a service-user decision and may mean moving on to a new plan or aspiration, or moving on from the service.

Walking an individual story through a traditional and a Social Model OT process

As a Local Authority (LA) OT, I was asked to visit a young man following a series of complaints from his neighbours (regarding the noise) and his home helps (who found him rude and intimidating).

He was in his twenties, and had had a serious motor bike accident a few years before. When I met him he was a wheelchair-user, he'd been re-housed in a council bungalow from the city to a rural village, his neighbours were all older people, and he had no job. He received mobility allowance, but he couldn't access the infrequent local bus. He'd been offered and declined a place at a 'work rehab unit'. He liked music – and played it loud and late (thus causing the neighbours to complain) and he resented his dependence on home helps and meals on wheels. The traditional approach had re-housed him in an adapted bungalow, sorted his benefits, provided home care, ensured he was fed and offered him an off-the-shelf solution to looking at employment.

We talked…all he wanted was for life to be accessible again. We talked through some of the things that might deliver this and eventually decided that the answer lay in driving. We persuaded the LA that what would really work was paying for driving lessons. Over the next couple of years he learnt to drive, got himself a Motability car, did his own shopping and cooking, went in to town for the night life, got himself a job and had no ongoing support service from the LA.

Applying a Social Model OT process to music-based activities

The language used is that of a journey, not necessarily a journey to some pre-agreed destination, but an explorative journey that stops to investigate things that look interesting along the way. A destination may only be seen as such on arrival (Oh yes, that was it!).

Information and invitation

Sometimes the people I work with are eager musicians, keen CD collectors and very clear that music is their thing. They may want to try out some things, learn some things and have some fun with it. Sometimes it's other people (often family or key workers) who know an individual well and suggest to them that they might like to try some music-based activities; sometimes the individual is excited by that idea, sometimes willing, sometimes resigned, sometimes reluctant, sometimes appalled…and my first task is to make the judgement call about when to push and when not to.

Many of the people I work with find trying new things difficult and avoid doing so. If, when I meet people, they give me any inkling that they might enjoy involvement in music then I do take time, I do persist and sometimes I do push and even strike bargains: I do whatever I need to do to get them to meet me halfway and give it a try. Sometimes I wonder if that's too powerful and controlling, but mostly I think that as long as I question that, then the extra push, support and encouragement people need to step out of what's usual for them is part of how I take responsibility for making the music accessible. Taking time to understand an individual's communication (see Intensive interaction in Chapter 5), to engage with them through their sounds and to establish a space for safe and open dialogue is often all it takes to make trying something new, possible.

Assessment/exploration

Assessment is about finding out where people are and walking their path with them. My role in that assessment is to listen to what's important to people, to understand what they'd liked to achieve and to work out, with them, how that can be possible. Finding out about people's favourite songs, artists or instruments is essential here too; it provides ideas and resources for intervention that will be motivating and fun. Assessment cannot be a one-off event; gaining knowledge and understanding and developing a co-operative working arrangement takes time. Motivations and aspirations change too. Sometimes assessment is organic and it's necessary to guard against it becoming covert too. Sometimes the working relationship benefits from the formality of stopping, taking stock and moving on. Using early assessment information to identify some quick wins can be a very positive way of building the confidence, excitement and motivation needed to take on more challenging opportunities.

Agreeing a plan

My role is to create an environment for success based on open-mindedness, creative thinking, careful planning and realistic goal setting.

Goal setting is not simply a case of realism. Goals are irrelevant unless they reflect individual priorities (playing a particular song, trying a particular instrument) and preferences (favourite songs or singers) and take into account individual satisfaction with performance (following COPM principles, see Chapter 5).

Goals may be:

1. Specific to the activity (X will play two different instruments during the music session).

2. Related to acquisition of musical (X will play a chosen song) or non-musical (e.g. social (X will make eye contact with one other person in the group during the activity)) or physical (X will get down to and up from the floor) skills.

3. Linked to a care plan (X will not scream during the session).

The goals I set with people mostly fall into categories 1 and 2: these are the areas where people are most likely to have a view about what they want to achieve. I do also agree goals in category 3 with people. These tend to be led by me and given in the form of a question (e.g. Do you think you can try and join in until 11 o'clock? Could you try not to scream whilst we record this song? Would you be able to sit next to X whilst we do this activity?). I have an awareness of what might be useful, in the broadest sense, and take opportunities as they arise. Pre-planned goals, linked to point 3, are sometimes agreed as a reaction to something that's happened over several sessions, particularly if it's something that is limiting or preventing the participation or development of an individual or the whole group (see Gavin and Popples' story at the end of Chapter 8).

The people I currently work with do not have written individual plans that relate to their participation in music-based activities. We have some collective aims; for the music groups these are recorded on the activity plan (see Activity Plans in Chapter 11), for the band, they relate to forthcoming performances, recording new songs and so on. I have some individual agreements with people about specific instrument skills they'd like to work on, or the roles they would like to take in the performance of particular songs. For me, to formalise our music into individual plans would be to turn the music we do into 'therapy'. I am not a Music Therapist and this is not what our music is about; our music-making reflects the view that music is an important human activity. The people who 'do' music with me choose their own journeys. I do sometimes write reflectively about what we've done and what we might do next. We do record and film ourselves so that we can track some of the important events in our journey. We do include some of the milestones in the lyrics of our songs. When I'm asked to give feedback to care managers, parents and carers, the feedback they get is this evidence of what we have done.

About process and outcome

Behavioural goals are outcome focused: they take a 'point in time' measurement of achievement. Sometimes, whether because of the individual's motivation or the nature of the activity, it's not the outcome that is important. Some approaches to learning (like Montessori) are premised on the belief that it's the process that's important, not the outcome. Some human occupations produce an end-product (e.g. cookery); some don't (e.g. going for a walk). Music-based activities may or may not end with a product (writing a song or playing for fun). One is not necessarily of greater value than the other. Value depends on so many things. As individuals we probably all vary in the extent to which we value process as compared to outcome. This will vary depending on the what, when, why and how, but we probably all have a leaning towards one or the other too. Some people are much more rewarded by the journey than the arrival (do you shop for the pleasure or the purchase?). If you have a strong pull in one direction you need to be very aware of it so that you don't impose it on everyone else (e.g. the well-meaning staff member who 'improves' people's art work). If the individuals have valued the process, it may be irrelevant whether the end result goes in the bin or on the wall.

About aims

Group session plans (see Activity Plans, Chapter 11) usually have a set of aims; some process, some outcome. An aim is not as specific as a goal. It's a broad statement of what I think we're going to get out of what we're doing.

Following the plan

Whether I'm teaching instrumental skills to primary school children, music theory to adults or facilitating a group for people with learning difficulties, the approach is the same: I do not have a 'special' approach for working with disabled people.

My approach will:

- focus on enabling participation

- use developmental models (for example when trying to work out how people's physical abilities, co-ordination, etc. can best be used to gain the instrumental skills they want to gain)
- make use of learning styles
- sometimes use adaptation and compensation
- engage people's motivation and enthusiasm by breaking down their favourite music to demonstrate and teach skills on their favourite instruments
- make use of many types of music
- encourage people to engage with music in many different ways (listening, playing, dancing, watching)
- offer one-to-one, band (ensemble) and large group sessions.

The essential ingredient for anyone who wants to develop musical ability is TIME – it takes a significant amount of time to learn, to find out, to try, to practise, to succeed (Levitin 2006).

About transferrable learning

There are non-musical benefits for anyone participating in musical activity; developing self-confidence and self-esteem, having a voice, experiencing emotions, trying out social skills, being part of a group, learning something new, etc. (see Transferability of musical and non-musical skills diagram, Chapter 8). These transferrable benefits are sometimes incidental. Sometimes, though, there is an opportunity to use music-based activity intentionally to develop skills in other areas (see anecdote, Developing instrumental and vocal skills, Chapter 8). If music is to be used intentionally as a means of working on other things this should be declared, discussed, chosen and agreed, never covert.

Talking about how it's going and moving on

The evaluation of individual achievements belongs to the individual. Following the COPM framework (see Chapter 5) can provide useful feedback to the individual about what they have achieved and what they'd like to focus on next.

Service evaluation focuses on the accessibility of the service. I write notes and reflections after each session so that I can think about what is happening. I use holidays, often, as a check point: a time to stop, appraise, re-focus and plan for the future. I get a big buzz from seeing how people flourish in an encouraging and accessible environment and I think it's important to acknowledge that: what I do isn't self-less, it makes me feel good.

The musical performances both in the groups and in the band are never 'propped up' by professional musicians: The Band are The Band. They have come an incredible distance in a very short time and are still travelling. Their performances are significantly better than 'good enough'. For me, one of the important things about working with people with learning difficulties is wanting the people who see or hear them play to say, 'Wow, that was amazing' or 'Actually, I think that still needs a bit of work,' not 'Ah, it's nice to see them having fun.' Well-meaning, disingenuous praise is disabling. They have a right to receive honest and respectful feedback. They will not become perceptive self-critics without that. Where performance is involved one of my tasks with band members is, having ensured I've understood what role they want to have, to do everything I can to make that possible and to be entirely honest with them that their performance has to be of an acceptable standard for them to be the one that takes that role.

Moving on

When you set out on a journey with someone you might not know where your destination is but sometimes you do need to remember what you're aiming for. I get very involved in writing songs and performing with The Band. Sometimes I need to remind myself to do less as they gain confidence and skills. I am the only band member that gets paid for being there; we have unequal positions and, whilst that feels uncomfortable sometimes, perhaps that's how it has to be until we have travelled a bit further. Ultimately The Band will know that they can do it without me and they may or may not invite me to continue to join them.

CHAPTER 7

Creating an Enabling Environment

The title of this chapter (see Swain *et al.* 1993) is a reflection of the assertion that the *impact* of impairment – the thing we call *disability* – is significantly reduced if we *all* take responsibility for creating enabling environments.

Being active and having a purpose is an essential part of the human condition. Activity gives us structure, helps define who we are, and prevents boredom, frustration, anxiety and depression. Everyone has the need to engage in activity, but people with impairments may have much less opportunity to do so. Enabling participation in activities by adapting environments and occupations can start to re-dress the cumulative, disabling effect of that reduced opportunity.

People First, an organisation run by and for people who have been labelled by society as being 'people with learning difficulties' is clear that such people can become more independent if given good support (see Web References). It is not that people with learning difficulties cannot learn, they may just need to do so differently from other people. The label, in itself, gives no information about the nature of that difference. The degree to which it is useful (or not) and respectful (or not) to have knowledge of people's history, impairments and diagnostic label is therefore debatable. In practice, applying the principle of approaching intervention with an open mind often serves well. The traditional OT approach to assessment and history-taking is arguably intrusive, disrespectful and unnecessary: worse still is a covert assessment disguised as an informal 'chat'. Sometimes history-taking and the use of diagnostic labels is a necessary part of a process (for example when establishing eligibility for benefits or insurance payouts) but perhaps the fact that it is necessary here is more a reflection on the inappropriateness of the system than the validity of the approach. It's sometimes incredibly valuable to have enough clues about someone that intervention starts with some best guesses about what's likely to work (see Reflective Practice and clinical reasoning in Chapter 5). It's so important to gain people's trust and it's so much easier to establish it if your early interactions are a success (see Conscious use of self and Intensive interaction in Chapter 5). In view of this debate this chapter sets out both general principles about creating enabling environments and some that are more specific to people with particular impairments. The intention is not to encourage pigeon-holing but rather to share experience that might be useful in ensuring that interactions with people are positive.

The role of legislation and social policy in contributing to the creation of enabling environments

At any point in time a range of social care policy initiatives are a priority. They are principally driven by central government and are often a reaction to either an emerging trend (e.g. the moving and handling regulations that were the result of the growing number of care workers seeking compensation for back injuries) or a high profile story (e.g. the endemic abuse found in a named residential home). They are written with the intention of addressing the issues that have been raised and sometimes have a very positive impact. Sometimes, though, rushed or 'one size fits all' implementation and the imposition of blunt performance indicators may lead to a less enabling individual experience than the one that was intended.

Normalisation and age appropriateness

The principle of normalisation was first articulated in the late 1960s and strongly influenced policy development across the world in the 1970s and 1980s. The principle did not mean that 'People with learning difficulties should be expected to conform to the statistical norms of behaviour within a society.' The intention was to promote acceptance of individuals and improve their access to society (for example education, employment and social activities) (Culham and Nind 2003).

Despite attempts to challenge misinterpretation of the normalisation principle, it became widely unfashionable to use or encourage activities that the public might see as age inappropriate. As a policy initiative this usefully challenged some pervasive stereotypes (e.g. women with learning difficulties being dressed in ankle socks and having their hair in bunches) but it also prompted the demise, in some settings, of some valuable things, for example playing on the floor, giving hugs (which were replaced by handshakes) and using songs considered childish (nursery rhymes).

I was once told a story by a support worker of a young woman who had always had a nursery rhyme tape on at bedtime. It was deemed age inappropriate and stopped. She screamed and became very distressed by any attempt to replace her tape with 'appropriate' music so no bedtime music was offered. She became 'challenging' at night…

A few thoughts about why nursery rhymes are where people feel comfortable:

- Singing nursery rhymes to small children is very natural; singing this week's best selling single to an adult child with learning difficulties may not be. Nursery rhymes are more likely to be familiar to adults whose independent access to music has been limited.

- Music can be an object of reference. Nursery rhymes may be associated with home or a relationship with parents. In the above example they were associated with bedtime.

- The music of a generation is core to the culture of that generation (its dress code, its language, its aspirations). People with learning difficulties are arguably most easily accepted by their peer group when they are children. Nursery rhymes are the music of childhood.

- Nursery rhymes are melodically, harmonically and rhythmically straightforward. They are catchy, easy to pick up, often repetitive and usually written in bright major keys all of which makes them irresistible.

Working successfully with people, whoever they are and whatever the medium, has to begin from where they are and from what's important to them. If nursery rhymes are the songs that someone loves or feels safe with then they are valuable. The normalisation agenda did not provide a valid reason for removing them. There may be valid reasons for presenting alternatives (perhaps that the individual hasn't been given the opportunities to explore music and make different choices) but these should be carefully considered and offered. Where this is appropriate, exploration of new material might start with music that shares some of the musical features of nursery rhymes, for example, folk tunes, classical music (particularly the classical period – hence the popularity of Mozart) and easy listening popular music (for example Status Quo, Abba and Queen).

Health and safety regulation and risk assessment

The basis of health and safety law in Britain is the Health and Safety at Work Act 1974. In 1999 regulations were published in an attempt to clarify employers' responsibilities since many employers had failed to implement the 1974 legislation and were therefore acting illegally. This caused a huge surge in health and safety activity; employees were trained, risk assessment and health and safety monitoring systems were implemented, process and paperwork designed. The main requirement was the completion of risk assessments to identify potential hazards and put in place appropriate measures to remove or reduce them, where reasonably practicable (HSE 2003).

Providers of Health and Social Care services struggled with the idea of not only needing to ensure the health and safety of their employers, but also of delivering their duty of care to service users. Whilst this increase in awareness had some positive outcomes (the implementation of Manual Handling Operations Regulations, 1992 (HSE 2004) led to an increase in the availability of hoists and transferring equipment and OT practice regarding moving and handling became infinitely more sophisticated), there was a downside: suddenly nothing was done without the completion of a risk assessment. Taking people out, trying new activities and so on became more onerous, and staff and managers worried about liability and responsibility. Many ordinary activities, like day trips, support workers taking people home to their own houses, encouraging people to try outdoor pursuits and so on, stopped. We all take risks, big and small, with ourselves on a daily basis. The purpose of risk assessing activities in a social care environment was to ensure that risks were only taken consciously, particularly where the decision to take a risk was made on behalf of someone who didn't have the capacity to make that decision themselves. The purpose was not to stifle activity and opportunity.

Specialist provision

The provision of specialist services seems to go in and out of fashion and the reasons are not hard to understand. When people have particular environmental needs it makes some sense for them to be with people who have the same. Services specifically provided for people on the autistic spectrum, for example, can ensure a high level of support worker knowledge, structure, consistency, managed sound and visual stimulation (there are even autism specialist architects). However, it's a short step from this to the misguided assumption that people with the same diagnostic label have the same needs and aspirations and this is, of course, not true. In addition, specialist provision reduces access to the rich variety of human encounter that the rest of us take completely for granted and that helps shape who we are; it reduces social experience and access to the world.

Care in the community

In Britain, community care policy and law seeks to enable people to live independently in their own homes rather than living, through necessity, in residential care settings (Brammer 2010). In 1989 the British Government re-affirmed its commitment to enable disabled people to live as independently as possible and to fulfil their potential (Brammer 2010). The aims are laudable and significantly more disabled people now live in the community, but with research suggesting that 25 per cent of people with a learning difficulty live in poverty and 50 per cent have no control over their money (Abbott and Marriott 2012) independence and opportunity to fulfil individual potential must be compromised. In addition, service provision is still, often, off-the-shelf and access to ordinary community activities is still limited (see 'Music and the Social Model of Disability', Chapter 3).

Developments and changes in legislation and social policy, followed by considered implementation and evaluation of implementation are essential to the creation of an enabling society. A lot has been achieved, but there is a long way to go.

Accessible activities

People who are supported in a residential setting or through day services may well find that they are offered an activity programme. In a genuinely enabling society, all community activity would be accessible and activity groups for disabled people would be significantly less necessary. However, support to access activity would sometimes still be part of what makes it accessible and sometimes this support might take the form of experiencing the activity and gaining confidence and skills within an activity programme before seeking to participate in community activity.

The 'activity programmes' provided in social care settings take many forms, ranging from one size fits all through to carefully structured individual timetables to no structure at all. The critical thing about activity is that it needs to be meaningful to the individual. We all have an activity programme of sorts with some imposed structure (school or office hours), some standing commitments (walking the dog, picking the children up from school), some daily tasks (shopping, cooking), some chosen activities (exercise, hobbies, meals with friends, trips to the cinema, holidays), some spontaneous activities, and some periods of relaxation and inactivity. Setting out to create an activity programme which reflects all of these elements for a whole group of individuals is a tall order. There are bound to be compromises. It won't be possible for everyone to do exactly what they like whenever they feel like it and in reality, that's life, very few people get to do that.

A good quality activity programme is likely to have a backbone of time-tabled group activities, some programmed space for one-to-one time that focuses on specific tasks or activities and some programmed free time, relaxation and choosing time. Supporting people to access music could be part of any or all of these areas depending on the needs and desires of the individuals involved.

Structuring an accessible activity programme

There are a number of factors to consider when putting together or reviewing an activity programme:

- **Number of planned activities in a week**
  Well-planned activity sessions, whether group or individual take a significant amount of focused time and energy, both for the facilitator and the participants. A packed weekly programme of activities may look impressive on the wall planner, but may not lend itself to quality time and attention. It's essential to build in planning and preparation time and to be realistic about how much can be done well. Planned activity should provide a structure for participants that is enabling, not restricting or over-whelming.

- **Range of activities available**
  There are many interest checklists available (see the MOHO website in the Web References list, or search for 'interests checklists' on the internet) and these can be useful in ensuring that the range of activities offered caters for the widest range of interests and aspirations. Regular taster sessions of new activities can provide a means of giving people the experience they need to make informed choices about the activities they participate in.

- **Best time of the day or week for each activity**
  Existing routines may impose some time constraints (for example transport times, specific break times for cigarettes, medication, toileting, etc.). Ensuring that the structured plan leaves enough flexibility around these times that they are not anxiety provoking or distracting (What time's the transport coming? When can I have my fag?). This gives people a better chance of being able to focus and concentrate.
  Everyone's energy levels vary naturally through the day (the sleepy after lunch slot being particularly notorious). It makes sense to schedule sessions at a time of day when they're most likely to succeed (a session requiring energy and concentration may be best timed for mid-morning).

- **Group and individual sessions**
  A balanced programme will probably include a variety of group and individual sessions for each person and part of the benefit of each session will be as much about this as about the activity. Group activities have all the potential gains of group work (see Group processes in Chapter 5), individual sessions allow a much more specific tailoring of the activity to

meet the needs and aspirations of the individual (see Chapters 10 and 11). Supported individual time for free choice activities and for relaxation is essential; everyone needs down time too.

- **Be prepared!**
  Good social contact and engagement in an activity can be easily lost and very hard to re-establish. Plan an activity in writing and make a list of everything needed (resources) to complete it (e.g. if you have to go to the cupboard to get something or if you don't have the right materials to make the activity a success). Sometimes an activity just doesn't seem to work or is completed more quickly than expected. Always have some contingency activities planned in case they are needed (see Chapter 10).

- **Interruption**
  Attention and focus is quickly lost, for example, by someone coming into the room with a message or by support staff leaving their mobile phones on. Unnecessary interruption is disrespectful to the participants of an activity and, other than in an emergency, should be avoided.

- **Duration**
  Twenty minutes is often cited as the maximum length of time most people can maintain attention. Activities or group sessions that last longer should be broken into manageable chunks with planned breaks. In addition, any activity has to accommodate people choosing to come and go. Frequent pauses can enable people to leave or re-join the activity with minimum disruption.

- **Group size**
  In a group setting people are more likely to get their individual needs met in small, well-supported groups. A group of six to eight is large enough to gain social experience and benefit from 'group' dynamics. Support staff are group members; if they are in the room they should be fully involved in contributing both to the activity and to the dynamics of the group.

- **Group mix**
  Inevitably 'groups' include a range of people with varying needs, impairments, likes and dislikes. Sometimes there is a financially-driven pressure to lump everyone who, for example, 'likes music' into a single group. It's essential to maintain clarity about people's individual needs and aspirations, and what they gain and lose from being in any group, or a specific group. People, particularly those with little or no speech or independent mobility, can be inadvertently sidelined in large, noisy groups and it is not always possible to accommodate individuals with conflicting needs within the same group. It's better for people to have a short, focused

one-to-one support than to be part of a larger group where they can access little or nothing of what happens.

- **Environment**
  Poor choice of room can guarantee the inaccessibility of any group activity. Selecting an appropriate room should include consideration of:

  - Space: If group members are using wheelchairs and mobility equipment a room with plenty of circulation space is essential.

    The amount of personal space individuals need in order to be comfortable in a group setting varies considerably. Ensuring people have the space they need is an essential part of creating an environment where individuals can concentrate on an activity.

  - Access: Both to the room and to the nearest toilet facilities. The anxiety caused by negotiating difficult access to a room will affect any session that takes place in it.

  - Temperature and humidity: Hot, stuffy rooms are exhausting and people may not be able to regulate or easily communicate their needs regarding temperature and hydration.

  - Décor: It may be tempting to cover walls in art work, but the stimulation this provides can make concentrating on a task impossible for some people.

Minimising the physical barriers to participation

Seating

A pragmatic decision to leave someone seated in an adapted wheelchair can form a very physical barrier between them and the rest of the group. For some activities a wheelchair may be a good choice (e.g. painting at a table or baking), for others it's not (e.g. relaxation, dancing, socialising). 'Appropriate seating' is that which enables participation and has been selected by considering individual needs and preferences and balancing them against the demands of the activity.

Positioning

People who are unsteady in their movement or who are unsure of their own body shape and size will find it easier to participate if they feel physically secure. Sensory feedback regarding body movement and position is directly linked to the surface area that is in contact with something solid (e.g. it's easier to balance sitting in a chair than standing up); increasing sensory feedback will increase confidence. Chairs with arms are more reassuring than chairs without. In order to free up extremities for movement (fingers and hands, toes and feet), the larger joints (elbows and shoulders, knees and hips) must feel stable and safe. Kicking a ball is far easier sitting down than standing up. Positioning someone so that their elbows are supported on a table may increase their ability to use their hands (to paint, eat or play an instrument) (see Bobath, The neuro-developmental approach in Chapter 5).

Health

It's essential to be aware of each person's usual behaviour and to think carefully about the things that may cause them to behave differently. A cold or flu, a headache, a poor night's sleep or just feeling low may leave someone not feeling like participating, and this may not be immediately apparent particularly if they have no speech.

Comfort

Being wet or needing the toilet, being hot or cold or thirsty, sitting in the same position for a long time or not having sufficient personal space can all make concentration impossible.

Distraction

Noisy rooms, interruptions or an excess of visual stimulation (pictures, decoration) that is unrelated to the task may all make it impossible to attend to an activity.

Sometimes there are specific things about people's impairments that mean certain approaches to managing the environment are much more likely to lead to success.

Working with people who have sensory disturbances

We have six senses: touch, taste, smell, sight, hearing, and proprioception.[1]

Sometimes people have disturbed sensation. Sensation may be heightened (hyper-sensitivity) or reduced (hypo-sensitivity). A few people experience synaesthesia (where a particular sensation is experienced as another, e.g. taste is experienced and described in colours). Any combination of the senses may be affected and this will affect the way a person reacts to stimulation. In order

---

1   Proprioception is sometimes called 'joint-position sense'. It's how you know the position your body is in, even when you can't see it. Example: close your eyes, ask someone else to change the position of your left hand and arm – can you copy it with your right hand and arm without looking?

to be accessible, activities may need to be adapted (see Chapter 5, Sensory integration theory and Adaptation and compensation) to meet people's individual needs.

At its most severe, hyper-sensitivity to stimulation can be very distressing and experienced as very real pain. Sometimes people have extremely specific hyper-sensitivities (e.g. an intense intolerance of the texture of a material, the smell of a food or perfume, or the sound of a particular instrument). Sometimes people are just very sensitive to all forms of sensory stimulation and find it difficult, or impossible to screen out stimulation that they don't need in order to focus on the stimulation that they do need. With any activity, clarity about the stimulation that is essential to participating in it must be considered. It may be necessary to remove all but the essential stimulation (by for example, turning off background music, not chatting during activities, removing patterned decorations) in order to enable someone to concentrate on the task.

Hypo-sensitivity may mean that someone requires a huge amount of stimulation in order to stay engaged in an activity. People who are hypo-sensitive may have very limited attention spans and tend to fall asleep even during activities that others find very exciting. People who are hypo-sensitive may benefit from multi-sensory immersion in sensations that are relevant to the activity following the basic principle of sensory integration (Ayres 1979).

Music, used carefully, can be an invaluable tool in adding additional sensory dimensions to any kind of activity. Musical activities usually involve sound and proprioceptive stimulation; further increasing the level of multi-sensory input is straightforward. Prepare pictures to accompany spoken instructions, use Makaton to accompany speech, use tactile and brightly coloured objects of reference (see Chapters 5 and 8 for examples).

Multi-sensory stimulation can also be a useful way of involving people who:

- find it hard to concentrate
- have some sensory impairment
- need additional information in order to understand a task or activity.

It is important, though, that the stimulation is related to the activity and offered thoughtfully. It is a mistake to think that having a constant backdrop provided by the radio or television is a good thing.

If individuals have specific sensory issues it is useful to know this when planning activities. It's pragmatic to begin with low level stimulation and to remove as much unnecessary stimulation as possible, to observe reactions carefully and be ready to adjust what you do as you gather information about what works best for people. It may not be possible to meet the needs of people with very different sensitivities within the same group.

Working with people with visual impairments

It's useful to know if people have any impairment of their vision when you're preparing materials. There's a world of difference between not reacting to visual cues (Makaton signing, facial expressions, laminated symbols) because they don't give you the information you need in a way you can understand it and not reacting simply because you can't see them. Most people who have a visual impairment have some sight; it's important to understand if and how they use it. They may be able to access the information if they sit closer to the group facilitator; symbols may be more effective on a multi-media projector (MMP) where they can be much bigger; or a combination of tactile, proprioceptive and verbal information may be necessary in order to make an activity accessible.

Working with people with hearing impairments

Similarly, most people with hearing impairments have some hearing; it's important to understand how they use it. In addition, it's important to remember that the effect of and experience of music isn't solely about hearing it. The driving bass of dance and rock music, the resonance of live acoustic sound, the timbre of classic instruments like cello and saxophone are visceral, a whole body experience. The experience is maximised by enhancing vibrational feedback: listening by sitting on a wooden floor, or with hands or face touching the speaker and by having the volume up loud. Low pitches resonate more slowly and so are easier to feel.

Working with people with epilepsy

People with epilepsy, and their carers or support workers, are often aware of their triggers (space, temperature, excitement, drinks, light, tiredness) and this knowledge should be used to minimise the likelihood of involvement in activities leading to a fit. Sessions should be well-staffed with people who know how to both ensure the safety of the person fitting and manage efficiently any issues this may cause for other group members. The use of electrical equipment and lighting needs consideration; the flickering light from an MMP is similar to that of a television, and the image on screen is usually less intense. Stage lighting (when performing) may present a risk to some people (and not just for people with epilepsy, it can be pretty distracting and also get very hot) as can spectating at noisy, hot gigs with lighting effects; festivals and outdoor events may be an easier introduction for people who want to experience live performance.

'Challenging behaviour'

Sometimes people carry a 'challenging behaviour' label. In itself, like all labels, it means nothing; however its connotation is negative. Behaviour is the observable reaction to something internal (perhaps a thought or a feeling) or external (something someone else has said or done or something in the environment). Behaviour that challenges, challenges the observer; challenging behaviour is not intrinsically negative and should not be labelled 'unacceptable'. An appropriate response to challenging behaviour is to try to understand its cause and its meaning, not to seek to stop it in the absence of that understanding. The Intensive interaction view (see Chapter 5) is that a more appropriate term is 'distressed behaviour' (Caldwell 2008, p.33) and that this is a result of sensory confusion. Distress and the resultant behaviour may be reduced by removing the stressors (e.g. by lowering the stimulation level generally or specifically).

Some behaviour (rocking, biting, screaming) may be about trying to increase stimulation and seek more feedback. People with autism spectrum diagnoses sometimes refer to their repetitive behaviours as 'stimming' (Roth 2010, p.83) to reflect their stimulatory purpose. Finding ways to increase sensory feedback and reduce anxiety can have a very calming effect (holding people in a good, firm hug works).

Some behaviour is a request for attention ('Excuse me, can I speak to you a moment'; 'You're not listening to me' or 'I need something').

Music and emotion

Music evokes an emotional response and if music is the activity medium this should be anticipated. A single piece of music may evoke entirely different emotional responses from each person in the room – and just sometimes, these responses might be big, intense and painful. Some group facilitators advocate the avoidance of particular types of music in order to avoid distressing people. This approach seems ill-conceived in two respects; first it assumes that the facilitator can predict individual responses and that there is a canon of safe music, and second it implies that to expose an emotional reaction is a bad thing. A positive approach to this issue is to be ready, as far as possible, for whatever happens.

Being ready involves creating a space where:

- people have permission from each other to feel and express what they feel
- people know how to keep each other safe
- there is an agreed way to managing both the individual and the group if someone becomes distressed
- it's expected that if something happens for someone that is more important than the activity of the group then it will take priority over the activity.

Experiencing music in a safe and well-supported environment can be a positive way for an individual to learn more about their emotions and how they manage them.

Enabling participation in music is about bringing together three components:

- the music
- the individual who seeks to experience it
- the means of realising that experience.

People are all different and have their own abilities and limitations, aspirations and motivations.

Music is sometimes very simple, sometimes incredibly complex, but any form of music or way of experiencing music can be broken down and reconstructed in so many ways that music can always be accessible.

PART 2

Practice

CHAPTER 8

Enabling Participation in Music

Activity analysis and planning using an OT tool kit

This chapter looks at breaking down music to make it accessible (from listening to a recorded track to going to a concert, from trying out a keyboard to playing in an orchestra, from performing a favourite hit to writing a song) by using The OT Tool Kit (Chapter 5). This is not and cannot be an off-the-shelf, one size fits all 'How to' manual. It should be used carefully and reflectively in order to make people's individual, musical (and non-musical) aspirations accessible to them. A flexible, creative use of knowledge and skills alongside an understanding of individual aspiration is the value a 'professional' is tasked to add.

'Music' is a huge whole, made up of many pieces. Participating in music involves developing skills and knowledge across a range of areas. The areas described are all interrelated; focusing on one will lead to development in the others too. Developing skills in appreciating music will impact on the ability to compose it; learning instrumental skills will enhance listening skills; gaining performance experience colours the way that the performance of others is appreciated and so on. Whilst sometimes related development is incidental, sometimes it's intentional (e.g. I do listen to music with the intention of improving my own performance). Participation in musical activity can also lead to the development of non-musical skills and knowledge; developing performance skills can have a positive effect on communication skills; playing in a group or band can provide an environment for developing social skills.

These dynamic relationships are summarised in the diagram below.

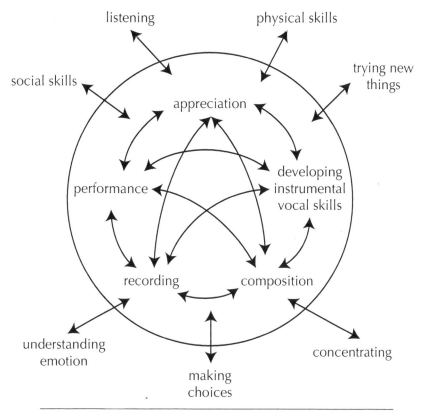

Figure 8.1 Transferability of musical and non-musical skills

General principles

A set of general principles apply to working with any individual or group and to focusing on any aspect of music.

1. It takes time

The value of time shouldn't be under-estimated. Any musician knows that time spent on focused repetition and practice is the foundation of musical skill. Research repeatedly evidences the 10,000 hour rule (Levitin 2006): It takes 10,000 hours to master the skills needed to become an expert in any endeavour – that's three hours a day, every day for nine years. Many people with learning difficulties have little access to music in childhood or adulthood and no access outside of structured groups. They are effectively denied the opportunity to demonstrate competence or expertise; they are not given the time. Time to repeat and rehearse the right things in the right way will always lead to improved performance.

2. Every aspect of music can be broken down and introduced a step at a time

Skills acquisition, regardless of the area of skill (e.g. physical, instrumental, social) can be based on a theoretical model or models (see 'The OT Tool Kit', Chapter 5). Analysis of the skills involved in a task can be used to build a picture of a developmental order for acquiring them; this can inform an approach where skills are built incrementally. The approach should not be prescriptive or linear; both the theoretical model and the developmental order will vary between individuals, between tasks and between skills. Any aspect of music can be broken down in any number of ways.

3. Music is an inherently multi-sensory activity

Music invites consideration of sensory integration theory and a multi-sensory approach (see Chapter 5). Whatever the musical activity there will be sound and there will usually be visual stimulation too. Dancing provides tactile and proprioceptive feedback; playing an instrument does both and often adds olfactory stimulation too (particularly with acoustic instruments – the smell of polished wood, rosin, metal strings, drum skins, etc.). When playing or listening to loud music the vibration is visceral. Music, in addition to being a multi-sensory activity in its own right, is a useful tool for increasing multi-sensory stimulation during other activities.

4. Music is adaptable

Whilst it may not be the first model to select, there are many ways in which musical skills can be adapted or compensated for (see Adaptation/compensation in Chapter 5). Whilst adaptation and compensation should not preclude the learning of a musical skill their usefulness, as a means of making specific tasks accessible and achievable, should not be under-estimated. A decision about whether and when to use adaptation and compensation should be informed by understanding, in detail, an individual's aspiration (e.g. does an individual ask to learn to play guitar because they want to develop instrumental skills? Because they want to play a particular song? Because they want to be on stage with the band? Because they like the sound? Or the feel of it? Or for some other reason entirely?). Understanding the *Why*, informs the *How*.

Music in an enabling environment

Inevitably music sessions can get raucous and noisy; it's important to manage sound, stimulation and distraction levels so that people can concentrate and relax.

Experiencing different aspects of music gives people an opportunity to:

- explore the components of music (see 'What is Music?', Chapter 1)
- feel the effect of putting them together in a whole music.

This chapter is divided into these sections:

- Appreciating music.
- Understanding music.
- Developing instrumental skills.
- Developing vocal skills.
- Developing skills in dance and movement.
- Developing the emotional and social skills of performance.
- Developing skills in composition and song writing.
- Keeping musical records.

Each section looks at the What?, Why? (Musical 𝄞 and non-musical ☺ reasons) and How? (with examples linked to 'The OT Tool Kit', Chapter 5). Where the model referred to would suggest a developmental approach the How? is set out in a developmental order.

> ...and personal anecdotes and examples are in shaded boxes.

Appreciating music

What?

Appreciation involves listening with understanding, both to the layers within the music (e.g. the role taken by different instruments) and the overall effect.

Why?

𝄞 Developing an appreciation of music not only increases the enjoyment of listening; it's a useful way of exploring different types of music and finding out about people's preferences.

♪ Appreciating how music is put together is an essential part of knowing how to take it apart (e.g. to do a cover version of a favourite song) and of developing skills in composition.

☺ Listening to a piece of music, whether recorded or performed live, involves a range of skills that are useful elsewhere. In order to listen carefully and not to distract others from their listening it might be necessary to sit still and quietly for a predictable length of time. Listening actively requires attention, screening out distractions, concentration and memory. These are skills that are useful for everything from participating in a conversation to going to the cinema and essential to learning, whether it's learning how to use the washing machine or how to sign your name.

How?

- Encourage listening by playing quietly and ask people to say when they can hear the notes. Play morendo (notes that die away) and see how long they can be heard for.

A sensory approach

- Start small – by using excerpts of short pieces of music. Focus attention by giving people specific jobs (for example – see if you can hear what instruments are playing, see if you can remember the tune, listen out for the really quiet bits).

Approaches to learning

Learning styles

Multi-sensory approach

- Play Snap: give people picture cards (e.g. instruments) and get them to shout when they hear it playing.

Shapes for prioritising

- Use pieces with catchy, repetitive rhythms and riffs (like Herbie Hancock's Chameleon).

- Use favourite tracks that people like/choose/ want to play/sing/are familiar with.

Motivation theory

- Introduce classical pieces by relating them to the popular pieces that 'borrowed' them: Procol Harum's A Whiter Shade of Pale and Bach; Greg Lake's I Believe in Father Christmas and Prokofiev's Sleigh Ride; the Wombles' Minuetto Allegretto and the minuet from Mozart's Jupiter Symphony.

Transferable knowledge and skills

- Introduce new things by relating them to familiar things; the ostinato (repeated background) riff on Can't Stand the Rain to the ostinato on Dido's Lament.

- Play Name that Tune: play the melody of a familiar song and see who can guess what it is before it's sung.

- Play chord sequences to familiar songs and songs sung in previous sessions and see who can guess the song before it's sung (see Shane's journey, Chapter 9).

Appreciating live performances

What?

Appreciating live performance adds a whole other dimension and an additional set of skills and knowledge both about audience etiquette and about how to handle being part of a large and often noisy, closely packed group.

Why?

♪ If you love music then not to experience live performance would be a crime; music so real you can feel the vibrations and the reaction of the rest of the crowd is thrilling…but it can also be quite socially challenging and frightening.

☺ Being able to manage yourself in a crowd of strangers obviously has other benefits. Understanding the etiquette, courtesy, manners of being part of an audience helps build skills for other social situations and is really useful in developing your own approach to managing your relationship with the audience as a performer.

How?

- Establish audience etiquette within the group: courtesy, taking turns, appreciating effort, giving space. Everyone knowing that if someone starts to spontaneously take solo time then the rest of the group will be quiet, give them room, listen and appreciate by clapping and complimenting at the end.

  Social skills development

  Group processes

- Set up the group room as a performance area with a stage space and audience seating.

  Social skills development

- Bring performances to the group. Arrange small private viewings, in familiar surroundings. Invite performers in as part of workshops (street dancing, song writing, belly dancing).

  Compensation and adaptation

- Arrange public performances in the group space that are attended by the local community.

- Prepare well to go to gigs and shows. Rehearse how it will be, watch live gigs on TV and on MMP. Think carefully about the factors that increase accessibility (will it matter where you sit? If there's an interval, if it's noisy, if it's dark?)

- Attend outdoor events and go to shows where participation is encouraged.

Understanding music

What?

Exploring the apparatus of musical expression (pitch, time, dynamics, tone colour, texture and form, see Chapter 1) by looking at musical form and musical meaning.

Why?

Understanding structure and meaning makes it easier to listen; it provides a route map for listening, playing and composing.

Understanding musical form

What?

Musical form gives composition a shape. Music comes in many forms and just as there have been changes in architectural style over time so there have been changes in musical form.

Why?

♪ The overall shape is important because it provides a map that makes it easier to follow the piece – a recurring melody or a familiar rhythm. Often composers set out to surprise and challenge by doing something unexpected with a familiar shape, but just as painting abstract art comes from a knowledge of how to paint accurate representation, it is necessary to understand how and when to break the rules successfully. Understanding form is an essential skill for writing convincing compositions.

☺ Much human activity, whether an everyday process like doing the laundry or going shopping or a social event like a conversation, has a form, a shape, and a process. Practising de-coding and following form can help make everyday processes more apparent and less anxiety provoking. It can also help to build planning skills.

How?

- Start with simple forms. Use folk and pop songs. Ask people to listen to pieces by focusing on one particular instrument or voice (try the Muppets' Mahna Mahna). **Approaches to learning**

- Sing songs and lay out laminated cards to demonstrate strophism (verse, chorus, verse chorus) and the idea of bridge, middle eight and coda. **Multi-sensory approach**

- Use singing in rounds to look at fugue. **Approaches to learning**

- Compare musical shapes to every day processes (e.g. cake form for sonata-form, having a conversation or a disagreement for jazz improvisation, see Activity Plan 5, Chapter 11). **Transfer of skills**

- Compare musical shapes to the telling of stories. *Peter and the Wolf* is a perfect starting point. The music tells a story but it's also narrated.

- Start by explaining strophism and through-composition and then go on to describe other forms and give examples – rondo, fugue, ostinato, sonata form. Ostinato is a repeated bass line. It's a really useful way of holding a piece together and there are some lovely examples (e.g. Herbie Hancock's Chameleon). People who prefer to do something repetitive are an asset in this musical form. It's also a useful metaphor for the dripping tap technique as a means of getting your view heard.

- Use examples to draw together the recurrent themes of convincing music: a strong hook, repetition, a definite beginning, middle and end.

Understanding musical meaning

What?

When actively listening to a piece of music, whether it's a classical instrumental or a popular song, the ability to find a simile or a metaphor is based on personal experience. The composer may or may not disclose their own influence but appreciating music isn't like de-coding a scientific formulae or doing *The Times* crossword. Finding a personal interpretation is valid and useful both as a way of understanding the music and of being able to communicate that understanding. Sometimes the meaning is an idea or a story, sometimes it's emotional.

Why?

 To increase appreciation and understanding. Music sometimes tells a story, has a message that's about ideas (programmatic music), or conveys an emotion or an emotional journey.

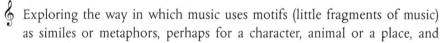 Exploring the way in which music uses motifs (little fragments of music) as similes or metaphors, perhaps for a character, animal or a place, and

the way in which music can tell whole stories by developing melodies for characters, blending the melodies so that characters interact, changing the mood with changes of tempo, key, texture and dynamic – is useful experience in deciphering and following code and being able to make sense of meaning.

☺ The world is full of code, spoken and written language and social signs (toilet, exit). As with any form of communication, understanding has many different levels. Most people have a basic grasp of musical meaning; a few people understand the language of music fluently. Developing the skills in music to understand simple coded meaning is useful practice for developing the same skills in understanding our coded environment. Few of us will sit down and read and understand every word of *War and Peace*, but it's very useful to understand the sign for toilet. Music can be used as a means of developing understanding about emotions in a number of ways and levels of complexity.

☺ People all experience a wide range of emotions related to life events – having a birthday, being away from home for the first time, making a new friend, getting flu, the death of someone close, the arrival of a new pet. These experiences can be used to give voice to and understand the emotion evoked by particular pieces of music (elegies, love songs, etc.).

Telling a story (programmatic music)

Sometimes the meaning conveyed by a piece of music is literal (Tchaikovsky's cannons in the 1812 Overture); sometimes it's more abstract (Mendelssohn's Fingle's Cave or Vaughan Williams' London Symphony). Literal music used as simile is easier to understand than music used as metaphor and so is a useful starting point. The simplest example of music as simile is the sound effect.

How?

- Play sound to picture matching games like Snap and Bingo. Use laminated Makaton symbols and Makaton signing.

    Use CD recordings of sound in categories (animal noises, machine sounds, human sounds).

A developmental approach – concrete to abstract

Approaches to learning

A multi-sensory approach

- Saint-Saëns, Carnival of the Animals — particular motives allude to particular animals. Put the animals on laminated cards. Play the melodies on CD one at a time and match cards to tunes, guessing which is which.

  Move on to writing your own.

- Set up Silent Movies using DVDs and multi-media projector (slapstick comedy such as Laurel and Hardy, or Buster Keeton) work well to start with because the sounds can be real not illustrative). Improvise the sounds for the film using instruments or everyday objects (see Activity Plan 11).

- Watch and talk about the effect on a piece of film of running it with different soundtracks and discuss the effect (see Activity Plan 11).

- Play pictures, photographs and paintings. (If this picture was music what would it sound like?)

- Introduce and listen to pieces that have been composed around the idea of paintings: Mussorgsky's Pictures at an Exhibition, Don McLean's Vincent.

- Paint pictures whilst listening to music. Use several pieces with different moods (Chopin's nocturnes, Beethoven's 5th, Tchaikovsky's 1812 overture).

- Explore pieces of music written for a specific purpose or to convey a specific scene like Vangelis's Mare Tranquillitatis and the Moon landing piece, both in *Music Express 5* (Hanke 2003a).

  Actively listen and then talk about what makes it work. Try out ideas and write a new piece of music.

- Listen to and talk about pieces that evoke a scene (Holtz's Planet Suite or Britten's Sea Interludes). Talk about the features of the music that make it convey the image (e.g. Holtz's planets – who was Mars? Would the music be high or low, fast or slow, percussive or melodic? Why? Britten's Sea Interludes – talk about seascapes and features of calm and stormy music.)

- Listen to and talk about pieces that tell a story like Prokofiev's *Peter and the Wolf.* Talk about the motifs and listen to them, shout when you hear the wolf coming (like pantomime).

Conveying emotion

There are a number of steps to conveying an emotion: experiencing the emotion, understanding it, expressing it, receiving it, understanding it. Music is a valuable medium that can be used for each step.

- Musical statues with facial expressions – the music stops; you stand still and make a face at someone else in response to an instruction (sign, symbol and spoken to maximise the information available and also give the opportunity for people who understand one kind of code to transfer their learning to another). Start with primary emotions (happy, sad, angry, afraid) and move on to secondary emotions (surprised, bored, anxious). It's fun but it also gives people an opportunity to experiment with their facial expressions and to see the ones other people use. (It can be quite an instructive way of learning how to read people whose facial expressions for particular feelings may be very different from your own.)

A developmental approach – concrete to abstract

Transfer of learning

Theory of mind (TOM)

Motivation – learning while having fun

- If people struggle to respond to emotion words or signs (happy, angry, etc.), use scenarios instead (the face you make when someone just gave you a present, or your swimming trip has just been cancelled, or you're going to a party, etc.).

TOM

- Play 'in the style of' musical charades (how would you play if you were angry?). Encourage people to choose both the instrument and how they would play it. Encourage people to guess what each other are expressing and to add their own ideas.

Conscious use of self

- Use the same expression cards as a conducting tool with people changing the manner of their playing as a piece unfolds and different expression symbols are held up.

- Listen to music and discuss and compare the feelings it elicits ('discussion' doesn't need to be verbal: it can be drawn, painted, danced). Observe people's reactions to different moods in music and question assumptions about how people express how they're feeling.

Clinical reasoning

- Use metaphor to describe emotions (what picture does this music paint?). Metaphor can be a useful way of arriving at a description that can then be related back to a feeling word, giving people additional information about the feeling that each feeling word is ascribed to. However, some people cannot understand metaphor, and ultimately no one knows that the feeling we each ascribe to a descriptive word is the same feeling (we don't know that we're feeling the same thing), so there are no right answers. The importance is in people being confident about how to communicate their emotions.

Group processes

- Encourage people to understand their own reactions to music. (Is there a type of music that cheers you up when you're low? That calms you down when you're anxious? That helps you to relax or to sleep?)

- Demonstrate how music can be a tool to manage mood (Roberts 2004). People in group sessions seem to react very rapidly to the mood of others in the room; sometimes there's a real flatness, sometimes tension, sometimes pleasure, sometimes excitement. When using music as a medium it's important that you pick up on and respond to mood throughout a session. Adding energising sound to an already buzzing room can be a disaster, using music to relax an already flat room is no more useful. Know your material and be ready to change direction.

Developing instrumental and vocal skills

What?

Exploring the basic elements of music: rhythm, melody and harmony.

Applying the basic elements of music in order to develop instrumental and vocal skills.

Why?

 To support people in exploring and achieving their aspirations about playing a particular instrument, making music of a particular style, or covering a particular song. However simple or sophisticated the original, it's easy to take apart a favourite popular song and, armed with some basic knowledge of music, to work out simple rhythms, melodic riffs and harmonies that can be put together to do a cover version (see Activity Plan 4 and Appendices 2 and 3).

☺ To develop physical skills. The type of physical skills that develop through gaining instrument skills will depend on the instrument the person is learning to play. Playing a drum kit involves fairly gross movement of arms, at the same time as using one foot: co-ordination is important. Strumming chords on a guitar will involve the ability to place left-hand fingers on the correct string, in the correct fret whilst also strumming with right thumb or fingers. Picking out a tune on a keyboard involves fine finger movement. One of the things that often prevents people from developing co-ordination and finger control is limited core stability; finding a good sitting position (see Chapter 7, 'Creating an Enabling Environment') can be incredibly liberating in freeing people to use their hands.

I once worked with a man who had no speech and poor active sitting balance. He was very keen to drum and also to play the keyboard. Finding him a sitting position that enabled him to prop his elbows (at a dining table on a carver) meant he could not only instantly play both instruments independently, but could also play in time and was visibly excited by doing so. In conversation with staff it became apparent that he'd never been 'able to feed himself' – by applying what we'd learnt about positioning him at an instrument to positioning him in front of his plate it was immediately obvious that he both could and wanted to feed himself. Initially he fed himself finger food (sandwiches and snacks) but in the same position he was very soon able to manage a spoon too.

How?

Almost any song can be broken down into a simple playable format. Often popular music focuses on and repeats one specific component (a melodic riff, a chord sequence or a rhythm) in order to make it memorable. Choosing favourite songs provides perfect material for developing instrumental skills; take from each song its most striking feature and use it to develop a particular skill. Queen's We will Rock You demonstrates the power of a simple repetitive rhythm. Tina Turner's I Can't Stand the Rain demonstrates the effectiveness of a repetitive melodic riff.

Sometimes people get addicted to a particular song and find it hard to listen to anything else. Rather than play or sing it repeatedly with no focus or, worse still, refuse to play it, identify its most striking features and use it as material for learning skills.

Percussion and developing skills in beat keeping and rhythm

Why?

☺ Learning about beat and rhythm encourages us to listen to our own innate sense of time. Developing a sense of time is part of how we feel safe in our space. Without this sense of how time unfolds (the time between breakfast and lunch, the time it takes to make a particular journey in the car) the world must be a bewildering and uncertain place. There may be no evidence for this at all but the idea that listening to or playing a piece with a very clear rhythm (Ravel's Bolero) and understanding how it unfolds over time must have a mirror in life. Most people seem to be able to learn quickly about the pace of a piece of music, the length of an instrumental break and the right moment to begin playing again. Abstract appreciation of the unfolding of a piece of music must surely encourage an appreciation of other abstract concepts of time. (When is lunch? What are we doing next? When am I going home? Are we nearly there yet?)

How?

Keeping beat

- Stamp, walk, clap or rock to a piece of music with a steady, driving beat (4/4 time) (rock music is good for this try Queen, Tina Turner, Meatloaf and Status Quo). **Neuro-developmental approach**

  Have the volume up loud so that the vibration can be felt as well as heard. **Multi-sensory approach**

  Some people are very attracted to vibration and will press their ear against the stereo speaker just to feel it. For these people drumming what they're sitting on works; stamp on the floor or sit on the floor and beat out a rhythm with your hands or use Cajons (sit on sound boxes played with your hands).

Developing the physical and co-ordination skills to play a drum kit

- People often find it difficult to use hands alternately rather than simultaneously. Start with feet instead, especially if people can walk. Alternate use of feet is more automatic.

  Conductive education

- Keep time to a track by walking to it and then by sitting in a chair and stamping alternate feet.

  Multi-sensory approach

- Rest hands on thighs so that hands are moving alternately too, work up to keeping beat by clapping hands on thighs.

- If people struggle to keep time increase sensory feedback by keeping time with them on their body; drum their shoulders, thighs or hands.

- Start slowly (but not too slowly – the easiest time to keep is about 60 beats/minute – like a ticking clock or a resting heart beat. A very slow beat is as difficult to keep as a fast one).

  Mood music

- Use wrist weights and/or ankle weights to increase the sensory feedback experienced by clapping or stamping.

  Multi-sensory approach

- Move on to drumming with sticks only when people can keep time with their hands – the feedback is more direct.

- Use sticks to explore different sounds.
  Play the room: radiators, chairs (especially wheelchairs) and wooden floors all make great sound...

- Use digital toys that light up or move in response to sound to increase sensory stimulation.

I worked for two years with a young man who very much wanted to be the drummer in a band and, when we first met, was unable to clap in time. We worked hard on foot stamping (he doesn't walk) and clapping on legs, then him clapping whilst I drummed on his shoulders. After two years hard work he could sit at a full drum kit and play a 4/4 beat using snare, hi-hat and bass drum (both hands and a foot).

Teaching rhythms

Allocate words:

- Try out how everyone's name sounds as a clapped rhythm, try favourite foods, try playing 'cup of tea', 'hot chocolate with a dash of milk', 'coca cola'.

- Play the rhythms of onomatopoeia and descriptive words (crash, bang, rolling).

- Work up to playing cross rhythms and use them to build a whole piece; split the room into groups, give each one a rhythm – first each group play in turn, then two groups at a time and practise holding their own rhythm whilst listening to the effect of it with another.

- Move on to various combinations and bringing groups in and out. Try whole group changing rhythms – first all together playing one at a time and then swopping what each group plays. It's a good way to teach samba – and samba is one of the few places, musically, where I've seen people with learning difficulties included in a positive way.

- Use songs to demonstrate how beat and rhythm can be used differently to generate different styles; most pop songs are written in 4/4 (four beats to a bar) (see Appendix 3). Introduce Bob Marley to see the effect of emphasising the second and fourth beats – reggae. Reggae plus a powerful walking bass gives you The Police. Try swing, blues, ragtime, tango and salsa. Describe these styles in terms of what drives them: are they rhythm, melody or harmony led? Were they written to dance to, to sing or to listen to?

- Use a drum machine or beat box to keep a steady rhythm.

Transferable skills: language to music

Multi-sensory approach

Compensation/ adaptation

Tuned and un-tuned percussion

- Explore the sounds that everyday objects make: play the room with drum sticks, make a band from kitchen utensils; set scavenger hunt challenges (find an everyday object that…); build on the everyday sounds that people respond to.

  Approaches to learning: behavioural approach – learning through experience

- Wheelchairs contain a huge variety of percussive sound – play the frame with drum sticks, run a stick around the spokes of the wheel; it rings like a bell.

  Playing it when someone is sat in it gives them plenty of multi-sensory feedback.

  Multi-sensory approach

- Use specific activities to explore sound – like making different sounds with water.

- Make instruments from scrap (don't forget to try wobble boards!).

Pitched instruments and developing skills in melody

What?

Melody is about the relationship between adjacent pitches (whether each note gets higher or lower, and by how much) and the duration of each note.

How?

Understanding pitch

Develop the ability to identify high and low and to hear the intervals between notes and to recognise higher and lower pitches:

- Understand the effect of pitch by experimenting with different voices, or with different characters (sing ten green bottles like a mouse, like a giant, like the queen, etc.).

  Activity analysis

  Approaches to learning

- Play with vocal effects – like sirening (Brewer 2002).

- Match a vocal or played pitch to a note produced by a digital tuner.

- Tune guitar strings to a tuning note by playing higher, lower like in the game show The Price is Right.

- Duel with keyboards: one person plays a note; see how many chances it takes for other person to find the same note on their keyboard. Start with a choice of two or three and build up.

- Use visual instruments (keyboard and xylophone) to reinforce the concept of high and low. Play them vertically (on their ends) so that the higher notes are visually higher.

Multi-sensory approach

Playing melody
Recognising familiar tunes

- Join in a song, or tune.

- Play Name that Tune and Snap (tune and pictures).

Play short riffs by ear

- Use familiar melodies or tunes with a repetitive melodic riff – the Muppets, Herbie Hancock.

Beginning to build a melody

- Use colour- and number-coded handbells to produce melodies made by the whole group.

The development of play behaviour: co-operative play

Social skills development

- Read familiar tunes from colour-coded music.
- Introduce unfamiliar melodies using a cymbala (see Activity Plan 2).

Compensation/ adaptation

- Some people have a natural ability to play by ear. Set up melodies using mirroring (play and echo back), call and response (question and answer) phrases or start a phrase and leave it hanging so it can be finished.

Approaches to learning

- Get the basics of instrumental technique right so that they can be built on (e.g. encourage melody playing with right hand at keyboard, encourage instruments (like guitar) to be held the right way round).

A developmental approach to skill acquisition

- Play with keyboard voices and unusual ways of playing instruments as a means of exploring tone colour, timbre and texture.

Instrumental breaks

Songs often have an instrumental break in the middle. The simplest way of structuring this is to maintain the harmonic rhythm (the chords used and the rate and order of chord changes) established in either the verse or chorus of the song and to play a composed or improvised melody over the top.

- Pieces written in C are a useful place to start. The Major scale of C has no sharp or flat notes (see Appendix 2) so improvising at the keyboard will sound great if the melody starts and ends on C and uses only white ones; the odd black note might well work too (see Marie's journey, Chapter 9).

Compensation/ adaptation

- Harmonicas and squeeze boxes are key specific, so as long as the key is the right one for the harmony (in this case C) any improvised melody will sound great.

    Chime bars, glocks and xylophones can be set up to only include notes that will work too (by removing the bars that have notes that are not in the key). It's great fun to play around with, gives instant solo success and really helps to build confidence to try other types of solo (see Appendices 2 and 3).

- Improvise over 12-bar blues chords in C (see composition below and Appendix 3). It's good practice and also a good starting point for writing a song (ref to The Colgate Blues (see Appendix 1 for lyrics and how to download the recorded song)).

CHOOSING AN INSTRUMENT

Playing any instrument well is difficult and takes huge amounts of practice. People play best the one they think they should be playing. Create a space where everyone gets to try everything and people will self-select. They may not pick the one that's easiest for them, but they'll pick the one they're prepared to invest in and motivation is what is needed. If they are physically unable to play their chosen instrument in the conventional way then work on finding a different way to play it. I try not to make any compensation that could negatively affect future developments in skill. And allow time…don't jump to adapt something that seems difficult – playing an instrument *is* difficult, give it time.

IMPROVISING MELODY

Some ideas about improvisation are described in the composition section below, but a word here about encouraging people to explore what instruments can do and not be constrained by conventional use. I worked with a young man who loved to listen to music and to dance. He had never been able to see and had no speech. I introduced him to some instruments, just by giving them to him and then sounding them in his hand. His guitar playing was amazing. Having never seen one played conventionally he drummed the strings and the body; he put it on the floor and slid his socked feet along the strings; he produced string bends by pulling the strings to sound them. It was fascinating to just sit and watch him explore the palette of sound that was available to him and to see how he experimented with putting the sounds together in different orders to produce his own music. It was also fascinating to see how long someone with reportedly a very limited concentration span was able to focus completely on a task that was entirely within his own control.

Exploring harmony

What?

Playing chords to accompany a melody.

Why?

♪ To make more interesting and elaborate sound.

☺ To listen, work collaboratively and contribute to the whole.

How?

A simple chord is made up of three notes (a triad).

It's possible to harmonise a melody in any key by using only three chords (Mozart did so to great effect).

The three most important chords, in any key, are built on the first, fourth and fifth notes of the scale. Any melody can be played or sung in any key (Happy Birthday to You is still Happy Birthday to You, regardless of the note (pitch) it's started on).

A band can perform knowing only three chords (and some very successful bands have been accused of doing just that) (for more information about keys and chords, see Appendix 3).

• Establish a colour scheme (for example D chord is red, G chord is green, etc.) and use it across all chord playing instruments. Use it to annotate chords on written music and lyrics too.	**Multi-sensory approach** **Learning to code and de-code** **Compensation/ adaptation**
• Experiment with right hand technique: set a challenge to see how many ways a string can be played. Listen to different styles of playing and demonstrate how the effect is achieved.	**Behavioural approach to learning: experience** **Kolb's learning cycle: learning by doing, listening, watching**

For stringed instruments:

• Use the chord colour to draw dots on chord charts and to put stickers on fret boards (play D by covering up all the red dots with your fingers).	**Compensation and adaptation**

- Practise right hand (strumming and plucking) on its own by open-tuning guitars or ukes (tune the strings to the notes of the chord so that no string needs depressing with the left hand) (see Appendix 2).

- Use coloured ukes open-tuned to their chord colour. They often come in the same colour bags – so the bag can be held up by the conductor when the chord should be played (colour matching).

- Use guitar slides to change chords and also to generate effects, without the need to depress strings on the fret board.

For struck instruments (glocks, xylophones, keyboards):

- Colour-code chords with stickers.

- Use a chord-beater (three pronged) for glocks and xylophones.

- Separate chime bars and put them into chords groups. Playing can be shared if necessary, each person playing one chord.

- For electronic keyboards there is often a function setting for sounding a chord by pressing one note (e.g. a D chord when the note D is played).

Compensation and adaptation

Developing vocal skills

What?
Exploring use of voice both without and with use of language.

Why?
☺ Singing makes you feel good.

☺ Sometimes people will sing when they don't speak. Singing gives a communication method and space to experiment with use of voice in different ways and to convey different things.

☺ Singing gives people who have some speech a space to experiment with fluency. The flow of a song can enable people who seem only able to speak single words, to sing whole verses. Encouraging strings of vocalisation in song must surely have a positive impact on the fluency of speech.

☺ The exaggerated modulation of tone when singing, as compared to speaking, encourages people both to listen and to vocalise.

☺ People's moods are easier to read if they're vocal about them.

☺ Singing builds confidence in delivering a verbal message and expecting to be heard.

☺ Singing can be used to encourage reading and signing.

☺ Singing can be used as a method of rote learning abstract information or lists (it works with the ABC song...but try something more useful, for example, singing phone numbers, addresses, name spelling).

> I've never worked with anyone who is completely silent. Sometimes people scream, grind their teeth, drone on one note...and sometimes well-intentioned support staff try to stop them from doing it. I work on the basis that we start from people's own sounds. Echoing back to people the sounds they make can be a very positive way of starting a dialogue that can then expand, in terms of range of sound, and can greatly improve understanding of the message that the individual's sounds are communicating (see Intensive interaction in Chapter 5).

How?

Without speech

- Establish some group rules around giving everyone time and space to contribute (so that airtime isn't dominated by people with speech).

  Models for prioritising Motivation

- Make use of existing vocal sounds. Use them as ostinato, build rhythms and lyrics around them.

- Explore music that uses vocal sounds (Adam and the Ants is good for this).

- Play with echoes. Follow rather than lead.

- Encourage people to take notice of each other's sound by sitting quietly without instruments. Encourage people to sing quietly enough that they can still hear the person each side of them.

- Build new compositions around people's sounds so that everyone has a part and so that group members echo each other.

- If vocalising isn't sustained use it sporadically within a composition or record it and loop it.

Compensation/ adaptation

- Sing songs to work on melody, pitch and modulation rather than the detail of language. Encourage projection and volume.

With speech

- Play vocal games (see Brewer 2002).

Developmental approach to skills acquisition

- Sing songs with vocal sound effects. Start with the familiar (Old MacDonald had a Farm; How Much is that Doggy?, The Runaway Train; Who Let the Dogs Out?; I Went to the Animal Fair) and use these to move on.

See normalisation age appropriateness, Chapter 7

- Sing missing word songs (Shout; The Lambeth Walk)

    And repetitive, rhythmic folk songs and shanties (What Shall We Do with a Drunken Sailor? and She'll be Coming Round the Mountain).

Approaches to learning: chaining and backward chaining

- Have solo time in the Singing Chair (see Creating performance opportunities, below).

Objects of reference

- Have volume duels: One, two three, shout your name the loudest – warm ups, sing songs with two parts.

    (Like Grease, You're the One That I Want).

- Sing in rounds (try camp fire songs).

- Encourage singing of words by using signs and pictures (see Activity Plan 10).

Multi-sensory approach

- Use songs that tell stories. Tell the story before you sing the song.

- Play 'Sing in the manner of…' (styles, emotions, famous singers – opera, and heavy metal) to encourage volume and colour differences.

A FEW THOUGHTS ABOUT 'SINGING IN TUNE'

Singing in tune can be encouraged by using a tuner for feedback, and by substituting voices for the guitars and keyboard head to heads described above; hear it, sing it , higher or lower? But…only work on it if it's an identified aspiration for someone.

My favourite track on the Wild Things CD (Sounds of the Disabled Underground Volume 1) is a song built around singing out of tune: it's a great song and the vocals are really impressive. It's called That's a Beautiful Thing.

Learning new instrumentals and songs

Listening (sitting still and quiet and focusing on hearing) is an essential skill for a developing musician.

- Listen to recordings of a piece.

Multi-sensory approach

- Encourage active listening by giving people specific things to attend to: separate the group into sub-groups to follow the line of different instruments, or give specific tasks (shout when the first tune returns or when a particular instrument plays).

Approaches to learning

Developmental approach

- Talk after listening. Encourage people to describe the journey of the piece (beginning, middle, end and instrumental breaks), to think about instruments they'd use to perform it and how they could give it a personal stamp. Use this approach when covering popular songs (see Activity Plan 4).

- Play along with recordings (fast tracks can be slowed down, without distortion using software).

- Divide the piece into instrumental groups (rhythm, melody, harmony, lyrics). Learn each part separately and then put them together to build the piece with either everyone trying everything or each person being part of one group.

  It's quite difficult to keep a part going when other people are doing different things; getting used to them separately first helps.

  Use a metronome for separate group practices so that everyone learns the same playing tempo (it really helps when you put the parts back together).

Activity analysis and a developmental approach to skills acquisition

- Learn from graphic score. A graphic score is a pictorial representation of a piece. It can be whatever shape the composer wants it to be. Its job, as with any musical score, is to convey to the performer the composer's intentions. Different instruments and different ways of playing them may have different colours or patterns (see Activity Plan 5).

  The shape of the piece may be represented by the journey across the page. It's easy to create a graphic score to convey the message of either an existing or a new piece leaving plenty of room for interpretation.

Multi-sensory approach

- Graphic scores are useful for soundscapes where specific melody and texture and consistent reproduction are not prescribed.

- For pieces with specific melody, harmony and rhythm (e.g. songs) reading from some kind of score may be an essential aid to memory.

  The most straightforward is perhaps to record specifics in composition blocks (see Appendix 3).

Developmental approach to skills acquisition

- If the instrumental teaching system used is based on colour-coding then colour-code note heads on standard notation if needed. However, this can be a useful way of starting to read standard notation.

Compensation/ adaptation

- Use games (Snap, Pairs, Bingo) to learn standard notation. Many successful pop musicians don't read standard notation. Don't do it if it's not necessary.

Approaches to learning

- Encourage people to invent their own illustrative notation system.

- Focus on a tight start and end to performance. Be specific (will it fade at the end? Will everyone come in after a count of four? What will the dynamic be?)

Activity analysis and skills acquisition

Learning new lyrics

It doesn't always matter if the specifics of the words are right. We often listen more to the speech pattern and the flow of the line than to the actual words, but if it *is* important to get the words right try the following ways to remember them:

- Make laminated picture cards to represent key words. Hold them up one at a time or give each group member one; sit in a circle with them in the right order and point to each as you sing or create a PowerPoint slide show (which can then act as a backdrop and memory prompt during performance). Some songs lend themselves well to this approach because the lyrics paint a picture (e.g. Wonderful World).

Multi-sensory approach

- Use Makaton signs (Try Morning has Broken and Imagine).

- Use objects of reference (see Activity Plan 10).

Objects of reference

- If you're intending to learn material the group has written themselves then set out to use lyrics that are visual, descriptive and lend themselves to sign and symbol and use personal references and in jokes – these are the bits the people in the group remember...(see 'Journeys', Chapter 9).

Approaches to learning

Motivation: use of humour, personal events

Developing skills in dance and movement

Exploring movement and dance

What?

Dance is movement to music.

Why?

🎼 Dancing to different rhythms develops the ability to understand and play them.

🎼 It's a great way of experiencing different genres of music.

☺ Dancing has a positive effect on day-to-day movement. Lack of awareness of body image is compounded by reduced opportunity or lack of confidence to move to disabling effect. Dancing or moving to music is play. Adults sometimes forget to play and only move when they have to do so, particularly if movement is difficult. Dancing can be useful in increasing both awareness of body size and shape, and confidence in movement whilst having a good time.

☺ Music tends to have a forward momentum; it encourages fluid movement (see Conductive education and rhythmic intention in Chapter 5).

☺ Dance music is written to invite movement; it's a great motivator for people who find movement difficult or frightening.

☺ Dance creates a space to play with self-expression through movement. The dance that accompanies pop music is often quite suggestive and flirtatious; it can be a useful way to explore, talk about and try out flirting and coming on to someone (e.g. Grease, You're the One That I Want).

We once had a street dancer who came in to the group to do a workshop with us. He was cool and talented. He did a performance first with spins, freezes and jumps. The group loved the driving, bass-heavy music. He broke down each set of moves and invited the guys to try them. People who usually found it hard to get on and off the floor were confidently spinning on it on their tummies and back in no time flat!

One person who found any kind of movement a struggle and had frequent falls at home that he couldn't get up from, said, 'Jane, I want to do that, I want to spin on the floor.' I said 'OK.' He said, 'Do you think I'll be able to get up?' I said, 'I don't know, shall we risk it?

He span, he laughed and even [though he was] exhausted he got back onto his feet when he'd had enough and was incredibly proud of himself for doing so. I was very struck by how readily people could be shown how to get up and down from the floor when they thought there was a good reason to do so; street dancing should feature on falls management programmes!

How?

- Encourage any kind of free movement to music: from whole body to just fingers or toes.

- Try it sitting, lying or standing. Sensory feedback is maximised by working lying on the floor (the biggest body surface area in contact with something solid).

- Try movement in big and small spaces (see Darren's journey, Chapter 9).

- Explore body shape, size and movement by holding people and moving them.

- Give people the experience of moving fluidly by swinging them in a hammock, bouncing on an exercise ball, or spinning on a blanket.

- Use parachute, ribbons and pom-poms to create a feeling of great movement when a small movement is actually being made.

- Props (ribbons, pom-poms) sometimes enable people to move more freely by taking their focus away from their body.

- Use a big mirror, a window or fly-wire a camera to a projector so people can see themselves move.

- Try mirroring – working in pairs and copying each other's moves.

- Try hand-jiving, use Makaton signs (try Born to Hand Jive or Funk – Jamiroquai or Maceo Parker).

Everything we understand about movement can be applied to developing skills in dance

Conductive education and rhythmic intention

Neuro-developmental approach to the development of physical skills

Multi-sensory approach

Compensation/ adaptation

Movement reinforced by speech and sign (see it, say it, do it)

- Use action songs to reinforce movement with words and signs (Okey Cokey; I Went to the Animal Fair; Head and Shoulders; One Finger One Thumb; If You're Happy and You Know It...corny but they are good warm-ups).

  Multi-sensory approach

  Approaches to prioritising: engaging motivation – make it fun

- Introduce songs with set repetitive dances: La Bamba; The Macarena; Oops Upside Your Head; The Time Warp; The Monster Mash; line dancing, salsa dancing.

  Learning theories: learning through repetition

- Try ceilidh and barn dancing with a caller to shout the moves.

  Multi-sensory approach

Movement reinforced by costume and/or props

- Use costumes to create a multi-sensory experience and help people get into role. Try coin-covered belly dancing belts (great for giving tactile, aural and sensory feedback to movement).

  Find a leather jacket and shades or a circle skirt and a hairband to create the look and feel for a bit of 1950s rock 'n' roll.

  Multi-sensory approach

- Use props. Dance to Jump the Broom Stick with broomsticks. Some people find it really hard to jump, but it's easier if you have a physical reason to do so.

- Maypole dancing and dancing with a parachute are both good ways of increasing the tactile and visual impact of movement.

- Exploring dance styles (belly dancing, salsa, line dancing, ballroom, disco, ceilidh, street dancing, rock 'n' roll) by inviting people to come and lead workshops make them memorable, sociable events – give some background, have a map, dress up, try food and drinks from the relevant culture.

  Motivation theory

Developing the emotional and social skills of performance

What?

Musical performance is enacting music for an audience.

It comprises:

🎼 The technical mastery of the piece.

🎼 The physical ability to execute it.

🎼 The emotional and social skill required to communicate with an audience (the subject of this section) (Rink 2006; Bonetti 2006; Williamon 2006).

The emotional and social skills involved in performance include the ability to:

☺ Be on stage and watched by an audience.

☺ Smile and react to applause.

☺ Deal with the things that don't quite go to plan.

☺ Work collaboratively with the other people on stage.

☺ Focus on the performance, whatever the distractions.

☺ Manage nervousness.

☺ Let your feelings about the music show.

Why?

🎼 Music-making is often a social activity. Whether sharing music informally with friends or performing in a formal setting music is brought to life by good performance.

☺ Good musical performance is always the result of a lot of rehearsal, repetition and practice. Seeing the positive effect of repetition and learning to enjoy rather than be frustrated by it (see Marie's journey in Chapter 9) can be useful when trying to learn other things too.

☺ Key social skills are practised and developed in musical performance: being the focus of attention, communicating with your listeners, showing your emotions in a controlled way. In addition, for some people, practising these skills in a performer/audience relationship is easier than practising them in intense one-to-one or group social settings.

☺ Ensemble playing presents opportunities to learn about roles, about co-operation and about eye contact.

☺ The leader/conductor experiences taking responsibility for the performance of the whole group and being in control.

I once facilitated a Youth Music Project for people with learning difficulties. The group put on two performances, a year apart. My sister watched both and said that the most striking thing about the way individuals had developed was the change in their social confidence both on stage and in conversation during the interval.

How?
Informal/impromptu performance

- Use games to create the opportunity for impromptu spotlight time. Most games can be adapted into a musical game: Pass the Parcel, Noughts and Crosses, Musical Chairs, Snakes and Ladders, Grandmother's Footsteps, Bingo, Beetle drives, Snap – can all have forfeits or points that are awarded for the completion of a musical task (e.g. singing a song, dancing to a CD track, playing a drum, choosing a song, etc.).

  Put tasks on laminated cards (like Monopoly Chance cards so that they can be re-used).

  The tasks provide a low-key, quick and simple way of people getting some solo spotlight-time experience: the focus is on the game, so there's little pressure.

  Social skills development

  Development of play behaviour

  A developmental approach to skills acquisition

  Approaches to learning

- When working on any task (e.g. developing a soundscape for a picture, telling a story with sound effects, writing a TV jingle) divide the group to work on different elements of the task and then perform their work to each other, as part of the process. The pressure is reduced because focus is on the task and performances aren't solo).

  Social skills development

  Role play – rehearsing performancein a safe environment

- Build instrumental breaks into songs and instrumentals so that people get solo or small ensemble performance time that is heard by the rest of the group without having the pressure of a whole solo performance.

Practise exposure

- Set up activities for individuals to present their music choices to the group (e.g. a DJ session or 'five pieces I'd play to introduce myself to an alien' (see Activity Plan 1).

  Social skills development: role play

  Building confidence

- Explore being on stage, one step removed by using puppets and masks to be on stage using alter egos, or creating shadow performers with a projector on a blank screen.

- Do any music-based activity in front of a big mirror. It's a great way of getting instant feedback and people often really enjoy it.

  Models for prioritising: motivation

  Multi-sensory approach

- Use a fly-wired camcorder to produce a live multi-media projector show (people can see themselves real time and huge). Start by just running it for people to experiment with and move towards actually using it to show performance of specific skills.

  A developmental approach

Creating performance opportunities

- Make solo performance desirable by creating a beautiful space to perform in and giving loads of praise.

  Objects of reference

  Behavioural approach: positive reinforcement

THE SINGING CHAIR

Like a lot of the best ideas, The Singing Chair grew from reacting to what was happening in the room. Two group members were keen to take the seat next to mine – I had the guitar and the music stand – so I suggested that the person who was going to sing loudest should have the seat and share my music; the first person took the seat and sang beautifully. When the song ended we swapped who was in the chair – the next person sang beautifully too. Everyone in the group took a turn – and even those who make little sound rose to the challenge and were keen to take their turn in the hot seat and make the most of it. I decided The Singing Chair should become a feature of our sessions and should be the most beautiful chair in the room. We used a few metres of crushed purple velvet; each group member designed and appliquéd their own design onto the blanket – we throw it over a lovely squidgy leather chair and use it for solo time. The blanket has also doubled as a witch's cloak and a coat of many colours – it seems to have the power to induce singing when you're wearing it too; it's a beautiful, tactile, personalised object of reference.

- Practise performance etiquette frequently. Make it a routine part of making music together (always face the front, be silent and still until the performance starts, smile when you've finished and acknowledge applause). **Social skills development**

- Create stage and audience areas within the room. Practise entering and exiting the stage area, facing the front and focusing on the performance. Practise being an audience too. Everyone is unsettled by the unknown; role playing performance and walking through how it happens is good preparation for the real thing. **Behavioural approach to learning experience**

Learning to use a microphone

Be aware that some people will have aural hyper-sensitivity; the feedback from an amplified microphone is a horrible noise and can be very distressing.

Awareness of hyper-sensitivity

- Start by using a mechanical mic (a mic-shaped echo chamber that amplifies the voice without using an amplifier) (see Appendix 5).

- Experiment with a digital voice changer (again there's no amplifier) (see Appendix 5).

- Use hat and mic intros as an ice breaker (see Activity Plan 9).

- Experiment with a digital recorder (see Appendix 5). It has a built-in amp and is a nice way of people getting to hear themselves.

- Move on to an amplified microphone. Keep the volume low initially and demonstrate how you get, and therefore how you avoid getting, feedback from the amplifier. Cordless mics are ideal: no wires to manage.

Create performance opportunities

Work towards performing well-rehearsed material in a formal setting by performing informally as often as possible. Practice, repetition, and experiencing performing in different forums builds confidence, reduces nerves and leads to more engaging performance.

- Perform for each other and for parents and friends.

- Build in a performance slot to every event – fete, party, birthdays and stage time at festivals.

We sometimes use our performance mascot, Popples so it's easier for people to face the audience. (Popples has a history with us – see Generating lyrics in this chapter. We wrote her a song, see Appendix 1.) She sits or is held up at the back of the performance space over the heads of the audience. The people on stage sing and play to her, rather than the room full of people in front of her. She's one of our in-jokes but she also reduces anxiety and is an effective object of reference; see Chapter 5. People know what they are supposed to do when she is there.

Recorded performance

- Digital auditory recording and video recording of impromptu unrehearsed material is great fun, can be entirely 'in the moment' and a first step towards more formalised recording sessions.

- Production on CDs on a PC using digital recordings for events (fetes, open days, etc.) and presents (birthday and Christmas) can provide quick and professional results that give people a concrete way of sharing what they've achieved.

- Production of CDs and DVDs can become a bigger project that includes designing cover art work, writing up playlists, making decisions about track order and so on.

Approaches to prioritising: motivation

Leading ensembles/bands and conducting
Practise following

☺ Just as a performance requires an audience, leading requires followers (many of the audience and follower skills are the same listening, attending, etc.).

Practise leading/conducting

- Model conducting and then encourage group members to try the role (see shaded box below: 'Conducting, power and control').

- Start with giving and following simple instructions: stop and go. Good bands always start and finish together.

- Use a traffic light (red, amber, green) system with laminated coloured cards to hold up.

- Practise following stop and go instructions as a non-musical task by moving and stopping.

- Move on to musical statues, dancing and stopping with the music and signs. Both of these activities use whole body, and so give good sensory feedback.

Social skills development

Multi-sensory approach

A skills development approach

- Introduce a beautiful conducting baton as an object of reference and to increase the desirability of the conductor role.

Objects of reference

Motivation

- Move on to playing and/or singing and following the same stop/go instructions.

- Practise playing quietly and listening (one of the hardest things to learn about playing together is not just to get louder and louder).

- Invent, agree and add more signs to begin to introduce the subtleties of interpretation (e.g. faster, slower, quieter, and louder and happily, sadly, jokingly and so on).

Compensation/ adaptation

Approaches to learning

- Use words and signs, then only signs to introduce more subtle instructions (use recognised signs and symbols, like Makaton).

- If you use colour-coding for chords, use coloured cards (or flags, like semaphore) as cues to chord changes. It's not a very efficient way of conducting, but it's funny.

Multi-sensory approach

Motivation

- Use analogies as a means of explaining the concepts of colour (mood, nuance) and dynamics (volume changes) in music. For example, a car drive – setting off from home; getting stuck in noisy traffic with lots of starting and stopping; getting onto the motorway and screaming down the fast lane; coming off onto a quiet country lane and having to reverse a few times to let cars pass.

  Or a storm brewing at sea – start with a calm sea on a sunny morning; then the clouds cover the sun; the wind begins to rise; the sea gets a little choppy; the sky grows dark; it starts to rain; the sea swells, etc.).

- Use film of conductors both to observe and to set up on MMP so you can conduct alongside the conductor as a shadow conductor on the screen. (Disney's *Fantasia* and YouTube are good for this).

Social skills development: role play, modelling

Behavioural approaches to learning: experience

- In ensemble (small group playing) learn about counting in and rounding off, give people specifics so that people work co-operatively not competitively.

Play development theory

CONDUCTING, POWER AND CONTROL

It's fascinating to watch people volunteer and experiment with having the conductor role and controlling the performance of the group.

I once observed two people, one assertive and very verbose and one much more shy and with little speech, have a minor disagreement in which the first had control.

The same morning we practised conducting. The shy person was the first volunteer and used their position to re-dress the power balance by preventing, through signed instructions, the other person from playing a single note!

The accurate appraisal of personal performance

If people are expected to be mediocre, unable or incompetent and if they are benignly congratulated for action, regardless of its quality, how can they learn to be an accurate judge of their own performance? How can they become reflective about their own development? Why should they be people who aspire? Music is a medium where people can see what it's possible to achieve when they work out how to do it, they want to do it, they try hard and practise. In addition, a musical performance is never 'perfect'; it can be something to be really proud of and still leave the performer with a list of things they'd like to change and develop. Experimenting with being your own critical appraiser musically, must be useful in terms of becoming your own appraiser in life and has to be a much less disabling space to occupy than one where the mediocre is congratulated because competence is not expected.

Developing skills in composition and song writing

What?

Composing original works, whether instrumental pieces or songs can be approached in much the same way as developing musical skills, that is by breaking down the task into the components of music, looking at them one at a time and then building them up together.

Instrumental pieces will contain some or all of the elements of music: rhythm, beat, melody, harmony, form and any component of music (words or melody, rhythm or harmony) can be a starting point.

Sometimes someone just finds something they really like, or learns a new skill they want to use in a song, or has something they want to say in a song and we build a song around that component. Wherever you start the components shape each other in the making of the whole: It's Good to Know (see Appendix 1 for lyrics) started with an existing melody so the pattern of the words had to fit into it. Hi I'm Jamie (see Appendix 1 for lyrics and to download the recorded song) was written lyrics first so it's almost a recitative, i.e. the rhythm of the melody follows the speech patterns. The The Colgate Blues started with a 12-bar blues chord progression. Scaletrix and Stickle Bricks (see Appendix 1 for lyrics) started with a palette of chords. Onamatapoiea started with a tango percussion rhythm.

We ring the changes and start each new song with a different component: it helps ensure that each song sounds unique.

Why?

🎼 It's a great way of developing musical skills and understanding.

🎼 There's no performance licensing restrictions to worry about if you perform your own songs.

☺ Music is a powerful medium for getting to say what you want to say (see the lyrics of Tell Me What You Wanna Say in Appendix 1).

☺ It's fun and having fun is motivating.

☺ Writing an original song is something few people ever achieve: it's something to be very proud of.

How?

Instrumental composition

Rhythm

• Use familiar words (like names) to provide rhythm.	**Approaches to learning**
	Transferable skills
• Use the word rhythm for another song (see Activity Plan 3).	**Motivation (using familiar and favourite songs)**

- Explore the rhythms from different genres (e.g. samba, rock, reggae, rap, punk, club, reggae, swing, blues).

- Use a drum machine with style rhythms to demonstrate and choose the rhythm for a new piece.

Compensation/ adaptation

Melody

Any random process for generating a melody is a good starting point.

Multi-sensory approach

Approaches to learning

- Pick a scale or a set of notes; allocate them randomly to the numbers on a dice; throw the dice; write down the numbers/notes; play them in the rhythm you've chosen…and you have a melody.

- Use other random allocation processes: fishing for notes, throwing a bean bag onto a score board, playing darts or hook the duck (numbers on the bases). Save the bits of the melody that work, change the bits people aren't happy with. You'll be amazed how easily a melody writes itself once you get started.

- Experiment with different scales (see Appendix 2) and modes to create different characters and styles of music (notes of specific scales and modes are easily found on the internet).

- To give your melody a musical shape write the random notes onto a template that shapes phrase lengths and cadences (see Appendix 3).

Harmony

- Select a key that can be played using the chords people know (see Appendix 2). If the melody is being written first, use notes from that key to ensure it can be harmonised using known chords.

Transfer of skills/ knowledge

- Try each chord against the phrases of the melody and decide together which work best where.

  (N.B. Harmonic rhythm changes much less frequently than notes in a melody. Aim for chords that can stay the same for a whole phrase and use all the ideas above about open-tuning, colour-coding, etc.).

  Compensation/ adaptation

- Use a tried and tested chord progression as the start of the composition. Twelve-bar blues forms the basis of many pop and rock songs (see 12-bar blues template, Appendix 3). (Listen to The The Colgate Blues.)

- Encourage people to pick random chords and chord progressions by experimenting with what they like. The result may well be something much more interesting than mainstream pop.

  Behavioural approaches to learning: experience

  Kolb's learning cycle

Approaches to musical form

A composed piece will sound more musically convincing if it has a definite shape.

- Choose and use familiar everyday shapes and processes to describe and structure the music (see Activity Plan 5). Try: Making a cake, a trip in the car, building up the layers of a trifle, a Playstation platform game (with that little jingle that keeps coming back), having a discussion or an argument, growing a flower from seed, making a fire, doing the laundry.

  Any everyday process or familiar idea has potential.

  Multi-sensory approach

- Tell a familiar story (like *Peter and the Wolf*).

- Use pictures to inspire soundscapes (Britten's Sea Interludes).

- Use of software to build whole pieces (e.g. eJay) by dragging and dropping blocks of sound. This type of software not only guarantees success, but can be used as a teaching tool for musical form (the power of the main theme returning at different points, the idea of having an overall shape rather than keep adding new material, for building and releasing tension and excitement through a piece by using changes in texture, tempo and dynamics).

Compensation/ adaptation

Composing songs
Using vocal sound, without speech

Use echoing. It works particularly well in one-to-one sessions when the other person can be left in no doubt that their sounds are being repeated back to them.

Intensive interaction

Developmental approach to skills acquisition

- Start by just echoing back, even if the only sound is breathing (adjust rate and depth of breathing to match). Mirror whatever happens – it's fun and often results in a lot of laughter.

- Once the nature of the game is clear take turns to lead and echo and just see what develops.

- Record the echoes and use them on a loop as a backdrop to a composition (Audacity is music editing freeware that can be downloaded from the web (see Web References) and is useful for this).

Adaptation/ compensation

- Try beat-boxing. Use Human Piano (see Favourite ice breakers in Chapter 10) to experiment with vocal sounds people can make and then string them together.

- Try Scat singing – use recorded Scat (Ella Fitzgerald, *Music Express 6* (Hanke 2003b), The Muppets (Mahna Mahna)) to jam along to and to demonstrate what Scat is.

- Improvise Scat over a prescribed chord pattern (like 12-bar blues, see Appendix 3) and record for an instant original song.

- Incorporate people's repetitive sounds, words or catch phrases into songs so that they have a built-in solo or the others in the group share their lyrics (see Craig's journey, Chapter 9).

Generating lyrics

The hardest thing about writing lyrics is knowing where to start; any random approach to generating words will do.

- Throw the book. Chuck a book down and use random sentences or words from the page it opens at.

Adaptation/compensation

- Use blindfold and pointer to select words from a magazine.

Multi-sensory approach

- String together words using poetry fridge magnets. This approach can produce some surreal lyrics and give people access to unusual and descriptive words without having to think of them (listen to Lucy in the Sky with Diamonds). It really doesn't matter if it makes no sense at all.

Motivating by having fun

- Try playing with story cubes (see Appendix 5) – throw the story cubes, make up the story and use it as lyrics.

There are lots of semi-random approaches too:

- Play Buzz word Bingo. Generate a list of words on a particular subject (going to the beach) or theme (words that rhyme with 'red') and see if you can use them all in the lyrics of a song.

- Fill in the missing words. Tell a story and leave blanks to complete (It was a _____ day, I was _____ and decided to _____ then _____). For slightly more surreal results use this approach but play consequences (fill in a blank, fold it over, pass it on).

- Choose favourite photos or images and sing what you see.

The LA Buskers' first song – and still one of their favourite songs – was It's Good to Know what your Favourite Things Are (see Appendix 1). The words came from picture boards (with pictures drawn or cut from magazines). Each member of the group made a board with their support worker about the things they liked. Then we just sang what we saw. They chose to sing it to the melody of an existing song they all know well and really like. Using an existing melody allowed us to just concentrate on writing the lyrics.

- Inspiration from other songs. Use favourite songs to look at the type of things people write songs about, for example, Peter Gabriel's Kiss that Frog tells the story of the Frog Prince. Write a song based on a fairy tale (they lend themselves readily to songs because of the catch phrases…'Fee, fi, fo, fum' or 'I'll huff and I'll puff' or 'Who's been sleeping in my bed?').

Scaletrix and Stickle Bricks was inspired by Nizlopi's JCB song: it's a particular favourite of one of the band members and got us talking about memories of childhood. The lyrics are all connected to stories told to each other by the band and their support workers. We talked about how you create a song simply, so that it sounds childlike (see Activity Plan 4).

People with learning difficulties and the people who support them sometimes face challenges about 'age appropriateness' (see Chapter 7).

Scaletrix and Stickle Bricks is, in part, a response to that challenge: a beautiful, childlike (not childish) song about childhood, written in a childlike way.

- Use current events both personal (going on holiday, moving house) or in the news to provide inspiration for lyrics.

- Think about protest songs. There's a strong tradition of music and songs as protest, from Shostakovich to Ian Dury (listen to Spasticus Autisticus). Use song writing to give voice to the things people want to say.

Tell Me What You Wanna Say (see Appendix 1 for lyrics and to download the recorded song) was written exactly in response to that statement. We talked about things we liked and didn't like, things that made us angry, things we'd like to do. Then we chose two chord progressions, one for verses, one for chorus. I sang, Tell Me What You Wanna Say, and then the band took it in turns to speak or sing what they wanted to say, in response. Then we tightened the lyrics up to fit with the melody. The song was written in under an hour.

- Use writing a song to work through specific issues and working through specific issues to generate a song.

Gavin became very fixed on a talking, fluffy toy that lived in the room we work in; he couldn't look anywhere but at it, he couldn't join in a conversation or participate in the group. He and I talked about it and eventually banned it from our sessions. It now resides under the kitchen sink. We made up a fantasy existence for it and wrote it a rap song (see Appendix 1).
    Popples is also our performance mascot (see Creating performance opportunities earlier in this chapter).

- Produce lyrics by talking about and rehearsing things that might happen – driving a car, getting a job, living in your own flat, falling in love…

Pandora (see Appendix 1 for lyrics and how to download the recorded song) is Gavin's favourite song. It has great lyrics and was the result of a conversation we had about what it would be like to meet a beautiful girl and ask her to be your girlfriend.
    We'd been looking at Ian Dury songs and tried to write a song in that punk style. There's an Ian Dury song called Profoundly in Love with Pandora so our beautiful girl is called Pandora in recognition of Ian Dury's influence on the song.

Keeping musical records

What?

Methods of keeping ideas and compositions, whether written or recorded, so that they can be read, learnt, remembered and passed on to other performers.

Why?

🎼 It provides a means of tracking developments over time.

☺ It gives what happens status, credibility and a concrete product.

☺ It's so easy with today's technology to produce written or auditory accounts that there's no reason for not doing so.

☺ It's a chance to develop and apply IT skills.

How?

- **Graphic score**. Signs or symbols are allocated as a code for each instrument or for different sound effects; drawing the sign larger may indicate playing louder for example (see Activity Plan 5).

  Multi-sensory approach

- **Composition blocks**. Composition blocks (see Activity Plan 4 and Appendix 4) are a basic means of noting in the moment what's happening (a riff someone plays, a rhythm someone likes, etc.) so that it's remembered and can be returned to later. It's also a useful way of producing an aide memoir for performers without the necessity of them reading a complex language-based or notational system.

- **Colour-coded chord and keyboard charts**. The colour coding system for chords and/or notes can be mirrored by putting coloured dots on song sheets to indicate chord changes.

  Adaptation/ compensation

- **Standard notation with colour-coded note heads**. Standard notation with colour-coded note heads are sometimes useful, particularly for melody players.

- **Digital recording**. A good portable digital recorder (see Appendix 5) will cost a few hundred pounds; the recording quality is good and they are simple to use. Recording digitally allows immediate feedback (via ear plugs or amp) and with addition of a laptop the files can be downloaded and burnt to CD.

I've never met anyone who has absolutely no reaction to or an entirely negative reaction to involvement in music-based activities.

Trying new things can be pretty anxiety provoking…but music isn't dangerous.

Creating a safe, positive environment where people can experiment with their voices, their movement, their assertion, their co-ordination – whatever it is – where there is no dangerous consequence, where, in fact, the consequences are fun and positive and rewarding gives people the following messages:

1. Music is fun.

2. Experimenting with and trying out new things is safe.

3. I can be successful here.

CHAPTER 9

Journeys

Applying a Social Model OT process

The LA Buskers are a band that evolved from a music group that I facilitate. When I told the band that I was writing a book about working with people with learning difficulties and music and about us, Marie said – 'I want to write some things in this book, Jane, can I do that?' And I said – 'Yes please, that would be brilliant.'

In this chapter some of the band and music group members tell their individual musical journeys...so far.

How we wrote the journeys

We:

- sat around a table and talked and wrote things down; things we remembered, we liked, were proud of or wanted to do next

- asked each other questions: what did they think when I first arrived? What had their previous involvement with music been? What were their best and worst memories of things that were easy and things that were not?

- told each other our stories, described our journey so far, talked about our aspirations

- focused, broadly, on the music – but inevitably the music linked to life and life linked to the music.

Marie, Gavin, Cassie and Craig each drew their own Mind Maps of the things they wanted to say. Shane's and Darren's stories are told by me.

After each individual Mind Map I've written a few paragraphs. In part these paragraphs reflect on what they've each said and in part they aim to demonstrate the relationship between their journeys and the Social Model OT process (see Chapter 6). The pieces I've written are a snapshot, describing a point in time. They set out a blend of where each of them was when we met (assessment), what they wanted or want to do next (goals) and what they've worked on and achieved (intervention and outcomes). This process is not linear; there was no one-off assessment, no single point when we agreed goals. What we focus on grows, changes and evolves, naturally. It's essential, as the OT in the process, for me to be constantly mindful that natural evolution makes it very easy to do things without tangible agreement and to ensure I don't undertake ad hoc assessment, set covert goals or decide, unilaterally, the focus of intervention.

Anyway, here is what they said.

Marie

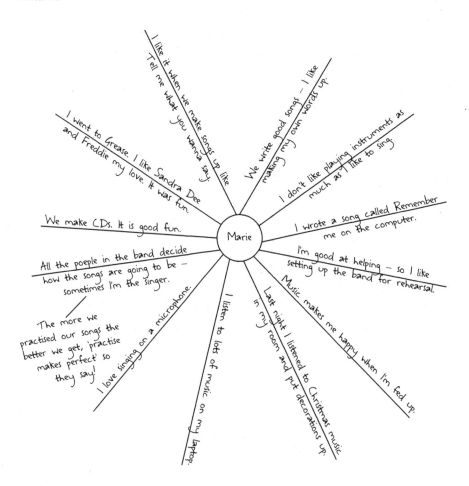

Marie is a great dancer and loves dance music. When we first met she was reluctant to listen to or play anything new, or to learn new musical skills and she wasn't very confident about her singing or playing. She gave up quickly and often said – 'I can't do that.'

Marie's love of dancing gives her a really good feel for beat and rhythm; she's turned out to be a good drummer. At the moment she finds it hard to sing and drum at the same time and when she has to choose usually the singing wins out. Marie has a confident voice now and enjoys hearing herself through the amplifier when she's singing with a microphone (mic).

Marie has learnt some guitar chords but doesn't like to play guitar because it hurts her fingers. If we need chords or instrumental breaks Marie is happier at the keyboard. She can play colour-coded keyboard chords. She can learn and remember short riffs and chord sequences and gets a big kick out of being able to mimic the original (Snow Patrol's Chasing Cars is a favourite). Marie has a great natural feel for mirroring the mood of a piece when she plays an improvised keyboard break. Usually we play keyboard breaks in C: Marie knows that if she starts and ends on C or G and sticks to the white notes whatever she does is great; she also knows that if she throws in the odd black note it'll probably sound bluesy (see Appendices 2 and 3).

Marie understands quite a bit now about the relationship between melody, harmony, rhythm and lyrics when writing a song. She's always very clear about what she thinks does and doesn't work and is very attracted to songs with a driving dance rhythm and songs with humour. Many of the lyrics of our original songs are down to Marie; she enjoys playing with words and making up stories.

Marie provides a lot of the band's drive. Marie can be relied on to make sure everyone turns up on time for a practice and remembers to bring their rehearsal schedule and song sheets and to stick around to help with the clearing up afterwards.

Travelling, going to new places and being in a confined space are all things Marie finds difficult. Coming in the car to see *Grease*, with the rest of us, was a big milestone and a measure of Marie's commitment to stretch herself. We had a great time and the knock-on benefits have been significant. Marie's working towards getting out and about much more and will be well-prepared for driving down with us to the recording studio to record the tracks for this book.

(Marie sings on Tell Me What You Wanna Say, The The Colgate Blues and What it Would Be Like to Be (see Appendix 1 for lyrics and how to download the recorded song)).

Gavin

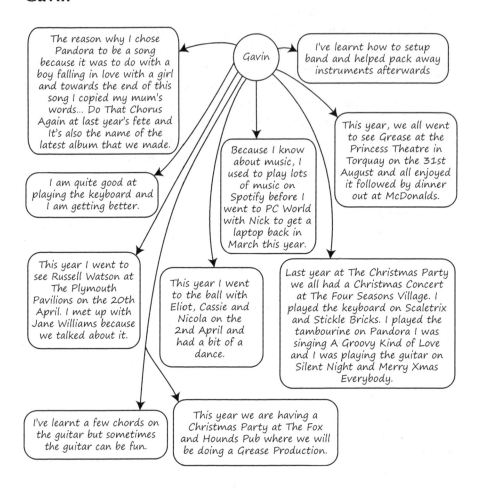

The reason why I chose Pandora to be a song because it was to do with a boy falling in love with a girl and towards the end of this song I copied my mum's words... Do That Chorus Again at last year's fete and It's also the name of the latest album that we made.

Gavin

I've learnt how to setup band and helped pack away instruments afterwards

This year, we all went to see Grease at the Princess Theatre in Torquay on the 31st August and all enjoyed it followed by dinner out at McDonalds.

I am quite good at playing the keyboard and I am getting better.

Because I know about music, I used to play lots of music on Spotify before I went to PC World with Nick to get a laptop back in March this year.

This year I went to see Russell Watson at The Plymouth Pavilions on the 20th April. I met up with Jane Williams because we talked about it.

This year I went to the ball with Eliot, Cassie and Nicola on the 2nd April and had a bit of a dance.

Last year at The Christmas Party we all had a Christmas Concert at The Four Seasons Village. I played the keyboard on Scaletrix and Stickle Bricks. I played the tambourine on Pandora I was singing A Groovy Kind of Love and I was playing the guitar on Silent Night and Merry Xmas Everybody.

I've learnt a few chords on the guitar but sometimes the guitar can be fun.

This year we are having a Christmas Party at The Fox and Hounds Pub where we will be doing a Grease Production.

Gavin loves music and can be relied on to know who sang what song in what year. He's an absolutely committed fan of *X Factor* and *Glee*.

Gavin has a great memory. I rely on him to remember songs we've half written. I know that if he's played a part once (keyboard, guitar or percussion) then he'll remember it regardless of how long it is before we play it again.

Gavin has learnt some guitar chords; he plays using colour-coded fret board stickers.

He can hold really tricky percussion rhythms together by learning them as speech patterns. He can play melody on keyboard, with two fingers (one from each hand) or play colour-coded chords with three fingers of one hand. We're working towards playing both together though Gavin finds this a bit frustrating.

He has a really good ear; if I sing a tune that's in my head Gavin can play it back to me (great for writing songs) and if I sing a single pitch Gavin can usually find the same note on the keyboard, first time.

Gavin loves to sing, especially solo (Gavin is the singer on Pandora). He tends to sing and speak with a very tight throat, and often lost his voice when we first met. We are working hard on producing volume for both speech and singing from the diaphragm. We're using singing coaching methods (Brewer 2002) and we're doing a lot of shouting!

Flexibility, spontaneity and imagination are difficult for Gavin. We've worked hard on:

- developing the idea of improvised instrumental breaks (when you've got such a good memory it's really difficult NOT to play the same thing every time) – listen to Gavin's harmonica break on The Colgate Blues

- inventing stories for lyrics: Pandora, an imagined love story, is Gavin's.

Gavin tends to concentrate on his own performance and has to make a very conscious effort to listen to, blend with and react to the performances of the other band members.

Sometimes Gavin and I miscommunicate; he prefers concrete, literal communication, I like metaphor, illustration, plays on words. Sometimes our miscommunications become the in-jokes of the band and sometimes they end up in our lyrics (Onomatopoeia, Scaletrix and Stickle Bricks, Pandora).

Gavin likes to write and draw and he also does media studies. He plays a lead role in designing CD covers and posters for concerts. It's to Gavin's credit too that we have much of our journey so far recorded on film and that we've produced one or two films to accompany tracks on DVD.

(Gavin sings on Tell Me What You Wanna Say, What it Would be Like to Be and The The Colgate Blues. He is the solo singer on Pandora. Gavin plays keyboard on What it Would Be Like to Be and Scaletrix and Stickle Bricks; he plays toms on Hi I'm Jamie and harmonica on the The The Colgate Blues and bass guitar on Pandora).

Craig

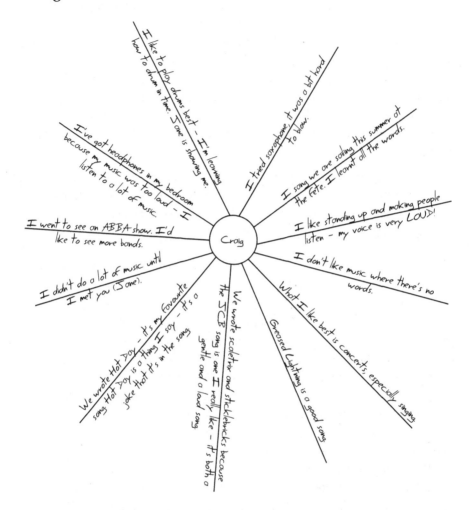

Craig is an explosion of energy. As soon as you meet him it is obvious that he loves to be in the thick of it, he loves to perform.

Craig will try anything and, though he might grumble a bit if it is not immediately easy, when he really wants to do something he will keep trying until he masters it.

The things Craig most wanted to do, when we met were:

• **To play guitar**. Craig finds co-ordinated movement and especially fine finger movement quite difficult. He worked really hard for a while, in one-to-one guitar lessons and can now hold chord shapes down if they are marked with colour-coded stickers. He's still quite slow at changing from chord to chord but he knows that, often, if you play a slow strum pattern with your right hand, you can create time in which to change chords. Sometimes, when Craig chooses, we open-tune a guitar or ukulele instead (see Appendix 2).

• **To play a drum kit**. Playing a kit requires both a high degree of co-ordination and the ability to get each of your limbs to do something different – it's difficult! We started by working on Craig's ability to keep time; initially by stomping around the room in time to music, then by stamping with alternate feet whilst sitting down – hands resting on thighs. I drummed beats with my hands on Craig's shoulders or legs. We did loads of clapping. We played Toms with our hands and when Craig could hold a steady four beat and keep time with a metronome we started using drum sticks. Craig can play steady, alternate beats now with sticks, as long as he both concentrates and stays relaxed. The key to keeping time is to relax; trying too hard tenses up your muscles and makes it hard to set up and maintain a steady pulse. Relaxation comes with practice and confidence. We're getting there.

• **To be the singer in the band**. Craig has a big, warm voice – we've used solo spots to work on singing, rather than shouting and on getting the lyrics as clear as possible. Craig can read, but finds it quite hard to read quickly enough to sing. He has made a big effort and learnt all the lyrics for the songs we're recording for this book.

Craig is a joker and brings huge good humour to the band. He's also a big fan of everyone else – quick to praise, to appreciate and to make sure people feel good about what they're doing. Scaletrix and Stickle Bricks was Craig's idea; he loves Nizlopi's JCB song (so do I).

(Craig sings on Tell Me What You Wanna Say, The The Colgate Blues and What it Would be Like to Be. He plays keyboard on The The Colgate Blues and drums on What it Would Be Like to Be.)

Cassie

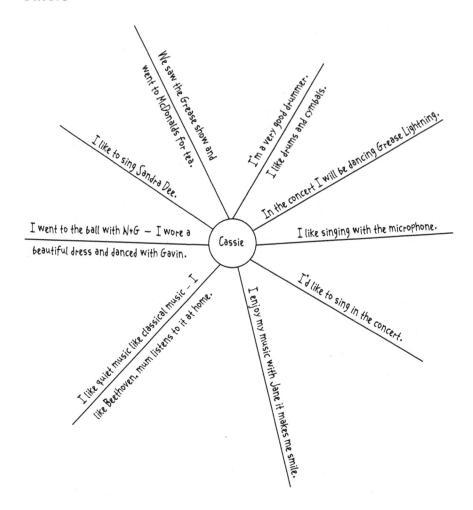

Cassie is gentle and reflective and shares my love of classical music. Seeing Cassie relax, close her eyes and drift off to the sound of Arvo Pärt (Spiegal im Spiegal) always makes me smile.

She loves to dance and to sing. One of Cassie's big achievements so far is to find the confidence to sing using the microphone.

She loves performance, both watching and participating and is a great mimic of voices and actions. Cassie really enjoys props, costume and make-up too.

Cassie reads well. She likes to sit next to me, when I'm playing guitar, and share song lyrics – she's an indispensible page turner!

Although she's reluctant to try playing an instrument, she loves the vibration she gets from strumming a guitar and she likes to use a guitar slide. Clarinet in its low register makes Cassie giggle and she loves slapstick percussion (hooters, whistles, slide whistles). I'm hoping to persuade Cassie to learn a woodwind instrument.

Cassie has recently started joining us for band practice and she provided a lot of the lyrics for Onomatopoeia.

Cassie is chief Makaton advisor on our song.

Cassie's careful listening and her determination that we will make a *nice* sound is a great asset and stops the rest of us from getting too carried away with just being loud and enthusiastic!

(Cassie sings on Scaletrix and Stickle Bricks and plays xylophone on Hi I'm Jamie.)

Shane

Shane has an amazing bass voice. His speech, in conversation, is usually in the form of single words or short clipped phrases. Shane's singing is confident and fluid; the words may not be clearly articulated but the flow of the vocal music certainly is.

Shane has a huge knowledge and memory of songs and will sing along with practically any genre of twentieth- and twenty-first century songs.

Shane is a great, loose-limbed dancer and loves to play air guitar. He loves to dance in front of a window or mirror. Sometimes we fly-wire the camcorder so that he can see himself projected onto the big screen in real time.

Shane is a natural drummer. In every group I've ever worked with there are a few people who just naturally keep the beat; tapping their feet or fingers or clapping. Give Shane drum sticks or a tambourine and the beat for the song is perfectly set up and maintained. Teaching Shane to play the drum kit took a couple of hours. He likes to drum and can play a basic four beat on snare, hi-hat and bass drum easily. The challenge for Shane is to stay on the drum stool for the duration of the song particularly if people are watching him.

In day-to-day routine Shane sometimes finds it hard to listen to what is said to him or to follow instructions; when he's enjoying music he listens carefully and learns quickly. He's been a great recent addition to the band – he works hard, concentrates for long periods and keeps really good time on drums as well as enjoying what we're doing and remembering the words to all the songs. It has been lovely to watch Shane become a core member of the band and to work respectfully with the other band members.

When I first met Shane music was fine as long as it was loud and there was plenty of movement. Shane found sitting still listening to quiet music anxiety provoking and distressing. Now he's a big fan of the quiet classical pieces and silences we sometimes have at the end of a session. He will not only sit still and silent for the eight minutes it takes to play Arvo Pärts Spiegal im Spiegal, but his progressive physical relaxation as the piece unfolds is very visible.

(Shane plays drums on Tell Me What You Wanna Say and toms on The Colgate Blues. He sings on What it Would Be Like to Be.)

Darren

Darren loves music; any music, live or recorded gets Darren smiling, laughing, hand flapping, jumping and clapping. He squeaks with excitement when I take my guitar out of its case and whilst he seldom gets up and changes seat unprompted, he will do so to sit next to me playing, especially if I'm playing loud! Darren has no speech and makes few vocal sounds. He chooses music by his reaction. It's very obvious the kind of music that Darren likes best; he is a glam rock man and loves Status Quo and Queen.

He loves to drum and will play long and loud for as long as he can hold the drum sticks! He will strum guitar but really enjoys using it percussively, by hitting it. When he wears it on a neck strap this not only makes great echo, but gives him lots of vibrational feedback too.

Keyboard gives Darren a chance to show his softer side, particularly in one-to-one sessions. He likes to play gently with individual fingers and explore different kinds of sound and voices. Where drums and guitar make Darren grin from ear to ear, his response to keyboard is one of quiet concentration.

Darren lacks confidence in his movement. He's unsure of his body shape (he walks stiffly with his arms spread wide and finds things like getting in and out of the car and going up and down steps difficult). Using movement and dance, particularly movement songs (Oops Upside Your Head, Okey Cokey, The Macarena, Lambeth Walk), give Darren fun time to explore and gain confidence in movement. Darren loves to limbo (which is great practice for doing things like getting in and out of the back of the car). He'll keep going until the pole is inches from the floor. With someone standing in front of him and getting to the ground as he does, holding his hands, Darren is not only confident to get to the floor but will squiggle under the pole on his back – he loves it, it makes him laugh out loud! Darren has a very acute awareness of when he's included in any activity and enjoys this inclusion enormously.

Darren holds his muscles very tensely and rocks continually. Music can provide a means of relief from this through relaxation. If Darren is sat well (both feet on the ground under his knees) and has pressure put through his shoulders or his knees he will stop rocking and flapping and become still; we sometimes do this with quiet relaxation music at the end of the sessions. To move and hold yourself tense continually must be exhausting and I'm sure Darren needs to have some still time. Sometimes we use a hammock swinging to gentle music; Darren loves this and will initiate getting himself down onto the floor to lie in the hammock to ensure that he gets a turn.

The goals I focus on with Darren are:

- having fun

- enjoying both listening to and playing music

- using music as a voice and as a means of expressing how he's feeling

- expressing his preferences

- using dance to encourage fluid movement.

We've all known each other for about three years now. Many of our songs, games and exercises have grown up over time. Our original compositions have in-jokes built into them and we are all connected by the learning we've shared in the time we've worked together; all of our musical journeys are shaped by that. The contribution of each member of the group becomes part of a whole. We are, in every sense, a group; everyone's 'special' and it works.

The LA Buskers have written about a dozen songs, we've performed at a few events; we've produced two CDs and a DVD. Five tracks have been professionally recorded (thanks to Owen at Dame Hannah at Seale-Hayne) to accompany this book. The lyrics for these songs are in Appendix 1 with web links for downloading the recorded tracks.

I'm ambivalent about my own role in the band; I love being in the thick of it but I am (so far) the only one that gets paid for being there and I do, usually, act as leader and teacher. I do take on the role of saying when I don't think it's good enough and I do prescribe what we need to practise; someone would do that in any band; it would be nice if it wasn't me and we'll work on that.

I'm incredibly proud (and I'm not sure that's very Social Model of me) of what the people in the band and the groups achieve. I see how hard they try, how much pleasure they take, how much confidence they gain, how much raw talent they have – they are amazing.

Memories I treasure

Collectively:

- writing our first song

- recording our first CD (including cover design, etc.)

- selling our first CD

- going to our first show

- all our live performances.

Individually:

- Craig singing solo at the Christmas party 2010.

- Marie dancing and singing the role of Sandra Dee.

- Cassie closing her eyes and sitting so still to listen to a classical piece and then looking up at me when it finished and saying – 'That was Beethoven.'

- Gavin grinning across at me when he'd just played an entirely improvised keyboard break.

- Shane telling me to be quiet because he was listening to a quiet piece and I wasn't sitting still.

- Darren getting down to the floor from his chair and bottom-shuffling across the grass to get to where I was playing guitar, under a tree.

CHAPTER 10

An Introduction to Music Group Sessions

Large group, small group and one-to-one sessions all have a place and offer different opportunities. In an ideal world the choice about the type of session would be entirely based on which is the best idea, but the reality is often more pragmatic. The flexibility to have all three allows the best use of the opportunities they offer.

TABLE 10.1 THE OPPORTUNITIES

One-to-one	Large group (6–20)	Small group (2–6)
One-to-one tuition	Social contact	Focusing on a shared goal
Easier to concentrate	Playing in ensemble	Developing relationships
Session can be tailored to specific, individual aspirations	Having fun	Collaborative working
Easy to set and to change pace, to change tack if the individual is bored or repeat as often as they want	Working co-operatively: taking turns, listening, having spotlight and audience time	Developing as a band
Focused time to learn technical instrument skills	Make good use of everyone's strengths to contribute to the whole	Individual can work on specific roles that contribute to achieving a whole

cont.

One-to-one	Large group (6–20)	Small group (2–6)
What's produced belongs to the individual, e.g. recordings, compositions or skills learnt	The rest of the group provide a trusted, ready-made audience	Changes in tack are negotiated, compromises are made by individuals in order to achieve the whole
Individual achievements can be practised and then performed for the larger group – good for self-esteem and confidence	The group generates energy	Space to demonstrate and further develop instrument skills
	People experience and can explore the musical tastes of other group members	
	Individuals can experiment without being too exposed – by taking one part in something everyone is playing	

Planning and facilitating group music sessions

A coherent group session cannot be entirely spontaneous; it starts with a plan or at least an outline. It is important though to feel confident that the plan can and should be disregarded when appropriate. As with live performance, sometimes a roomful of people buzzes with energy and whatever the plan the session is amazing. Sometimes it's much harder and the facilitator has to create the energy to get things started; the key to providing that energy is to be well-prepared.

How to structure a group music session

Regardless of the length of the session (whether it's a two-hour group or a whole day workshop) it can be planned around the same components:

- Identify some broad aims.
- Start with one or two short ice-breaker/warm-up activities.

- Focus the main body of the session around a few activities (two or three is plenty and linking them can help maintain motivation and coherence). These activities may be one-offs or part of an ongoing project.

- Build in breaks. No one can concentrate for extended periods. A social tea break has its benefits and can be a valued part of the session.

- Allow time to finish with a summary of what you've been doing and perhaps some ideas about what you'll do next time.

- Build in a cool down so that people go out of the session relaxed (sometimes the energising effect of music can make it difficult to stop).

- Always have contingency plans. If something just doesn't work or finishes more quickly than anticipated, move on to something else without the group losing momentum.

Whilst the plan is linear in shape it needn't be written chronologically.

Aims

Broad aims are often a mixture of musical and social. Sometimes they are a step along the way to a longer-term group aspiration (putting on a performance, writing a song, or playing co-operatively). Sometimes they will be framed around the specific aspirations of individuals within the group. Often they are simply about having fun and trying a few things out at the same time. They may be the last part of the plan that is written.

Ice breakers

Ice breakers are:

- a way to get started

- to put people at ease and encourage them to participate

- a way of saying hello, welcome, whatever you do here will be regarded positively

- short, fun, throw-away activities which last for just a few minutes

- critical to the success of the session

- a means of establishing an atmosphere and expectations

- easy and fun; nothing intimidating, scary or self-exposing should be demanded of anyone

- energising.

Ice breakers don't have to be:

- music-related; use whatever works
- the same every session. Repetition is sometimes good, doing the same thing every week isn't – who wouldn't get bored of that? If it is important to start the same so people know it's a music session, think about how you set the room up, use objects of reference (see 'The OT Tool Kit', Chapter 5) and maybe even use an opening fanfare as a call to arms.

The following are favourite ice breakers:

- **Action songs**: Okey Cokey; One Finger-One Thumb; If You're Happy and You Know it; Head and Shoulders; Animal Fair; Underneath the Spreading Chestnut Tree. And done 'in the style of' – opera singer, the queen, a spaceman.
- **Free-form jam**: just choose an instrument and play – play and sing, play to instructions (louder, faster), play along to a CD track.
- **Free-dancing**.
- **Playing word rhythms**: names, favourite Christmas present, favourite cake.
- **Camp fire and folk songs**: Ten Green Bottles; What Shall We Do with a Drunken Sailor?; Ging Gang Gooley.
- **Games**: Musical Statues; Musical Chairs; Grandmother's Footsteps; Simon Says.
- **Human piano** (people ascribe a voice sound to each hand, put their hands out, someone else plays the group like a piano keyboard).
- **Hand jive** (especially to loud funk music like Jamiroquai or Maceo Parker).
- **Mirroring**: copy each other's moves in pairs or in a group.

Ice breakers can be expanded to form bigger activities either in the moment, because they are going well and you don't want to stop what's happening, or for a future session (human piano became the basis of a beat boxing rhythm we developed for a song).

Activities
Sub-divide the activities for the main body of the session into types. This:

- ensures variety
- encourages development of skills across a broad range
- makes it easier to generate ideas and plan activities.

1. One-off activities

A self-contained task that can be completed in one session and re-used if and when it seems appropriate.

- **Games**: Musical Snap, Bingo, Snakes and Ladders, Noughts and Crosses, Spin the Bottle, Beetle Drives (see 'Enabling Participation in Music' (Chapter 8)).

- **Songs**: Break down a favourite, well-known song into lyrics, chords, percussion and put together a performance (see 'Enabling Participation in Music' (Chapter 8) and Activity Plans 4 and 10 (Chapter 11)).

- **Soundscapes**: Developing a piece inspired by a picture or a story (see 'Enabling Participation in Music' (Chapter 8) and Activity Plan 3 (Chapter 11)).

- **DVD karaoke**: Use microphones and multi-media projector. Make a stage, use costumes and make-up for a multi-sensory fun session.

- **DJ session**: Encourage people to bring and introduce their favourite music to each other – either in one session or as a long-running item where a different group member provides the music for each session.

- **Silent film soundtracks**: Use film on multi-media projector (MMP) to experiment with sound effects (see 'Enabling Participation in Music' (Chapter 8) and Activity Plan 11 (Chapter 11)).

2. Skill development activities

- Develop performance skills: Play games that focus on specific aspects of performance, for example voice volume (count to three and shout your own name as loud as you can). Establish a stage area and include walking on and off stage, facing the audience and acknowledging applause in solo singing time.

- Developing instrumental skills:

  - *Drumming*: One hand, two hands. Picking up tempo. Trying different beats (straight four, reggae and salsa) (see 'Enabling Participation in Music' (Chapter 8) and Craig's journey (Chapter 9)).

  - *Strings*: Open-tuning, colour matching, chords. (Colour-coded ukes and When I'm Cleaning Windows!) (see 'Enabling Participation in Music' (Chapter 8) and Appendix 2).

  - *Chimes and keyboard*: Melody, colour matching, chords, improvising (see 'Enabling Participation in Music' (Chapter 8) and Appendix 2).

○ *Voice.* Work on voice methods (Brewer 2002) use Singing Chair and solo time (see 'Enabling Participation in Music' (Chapter 8) and Appendix 2).

3. Projects

A large activity can be broken down into a set of tasks that are completed across a number of sessions. Working on projects can be useful both in providing continuity across sessions and in generating session ideas.

- **Putting on a concert** can include painting scenery, trying out costumes, learning songs, setting up the room differently, planning interval refreshments, designing tickets, sending out invites, writing a programme, doing advertising posters.

- **Song writing and recording** (see 'Enabling Participation in Music' (Chapter 8)).

- **Instrument making** (see Doney 2006; Thompson 2011).

- **Scrap band**. Create a band using household objects, found objects or things in the room.

- **Workshops**. Visit, or invite in people who do different things. Start off with a workshop and use this to develop a bigger piece of work. Try street dancing, belly dancing, salsa, line dancing, samba, ballroom dancing, Taiko drumming, beat boxing, handbell ringing and ceilidh dancing.

4. Summary

The summary can serve many functions. It:

- rounds off the session

- brings the group back together

- creates a space where things that happened in the session can be recognised

- can be used to plan

- cues that it's time to finish.

1. Sing a group song with spaces for individual feedback: Thank You Very Much works well (substitute the Aintree Iron for the things people liked about the session). Or just make it up: It's Been a Good Day (see Appendix 1) is a song we wrote that started as a session summary and grew into a project.

2. Recognition of something each person has done: clapping and congratulating or get group members to compliment each other

(either publicly or like musical statues – move around the room, when the music stops say something positive to the person you're stood next to).

3. Sing or play a favourite quiet song or instrumental sitting as a whole group (Love is All Around, Just the Way You Are, Killing Me Softly).

4. Make a visual list (words and pictures) to recount what's happened in the session and decide what to do next time. Agree anything that needs to be brought to the next session.

5. Cool down

A cool down at the end of the session can be used to:

• gradually bring down noise and energy levels

• give people who find it hard to relax a structured space in which to do so.

Try the following:

1. A parachute rippled gently by the group to slow music.

2. A parachute rippled over group members who lie underneath it, used silently and gradually brought down gently to lay on top of them.

3. Formal relaxation. Quietly talk through relaxation of different body parts one at a time to music or without music.

4. Sit still and quietly, listen to quiet, uncluttered music (minimalism is ideal for this: Arvo Pärt, Einaudi, Nyman). Use deep pressure and holding (see Darren's journey, Chapter 9).

5. Sit silently and listen to the sounds and silence in the environment (John Cage style).

Comfort and tea breaks

If the session is more than an hour include a break. A break:

• provides a non task-focused, social space and gives people a chance to interact in a less structured way

• gives the facilitator a chance to check out that individuals are OK

• gives everyone a chance to make themselves comfortable.

Contingency planning

One-off activities, skills development activities and ice breakers can all provide contingency material. A review of each group (see the stories that follow each

Activity Plan in Chapter 11) can be used to generate a list of activities that people have enjoyed and that don't require extensive planning and lots of resources. Activities can be taken from this list as and when needed.

Themed sessions

Linking activities into a themed session may help people to make connections and make the most of experiences (see Learning theories and a Multi-sensory approach in Chapter 5). A theme can also make it easier to plan and generate activity ideas. For example:

- **Celebrate an event or time of year**. Include food, music, costumes, pictures, films and making objects of reference (see Activity Plans 6, 7 and 8 in Chapter 11).

- **Create virtual journeys, e.g. a magic carpet ride**. Use a hammock, parachute or blankets as a 'carpet'; create scenery using a multi-media projector; choose your destinations by throwing bean bags onto a floor map. Then create the atmosphere of different countries using food, music and dancing, hats and costumes and essential oils or herbs and spices.

- **Build a sensory session around a song** (see Activity Plan 10, Chapter 11).

- **Build a session around a piece of film** (see Activity Plans 7 and 11, Chapter 11).

- **Develop a challenge**: Spin the bottle, or spin a dial and create sets of activities around the room or building (use headings, for example sing, play, listen, and dance).

- **Style days**: Build a multi-sensory session around a musical culture. Include costumes, food, dances and songs (e.g. rock 'n' roll: leather jackets, circle skirts, ice cream and popcorn, The Twist and The Mash Potato, Elvis and Chuck Berry, a juke box or a drive-in movie).

Knowing when to disregard the plan for the session
Sometimes:

- An activity engages people and takes on a life of its own (perhaps a ten-minute ice breaker grows into a much longer activity)...let it.

- A carefully considered, well-planned activity just doesn't work...put it aside and do something else instead; think about it later.

- Someone comes in wanting to do something specific...do it.

- Something amazing starts to happen in the room...follow it.

Facilitating is about supporting what happens, not controlling it.

Knowing when not to disregard the plan

Don't move on or give up too quickly. Learning and trying out new things, whether musical ideas, instrument skills or social skills take time. Don't expect instant success and don't be afraid to leave space and silence, particularly when encouraging people with little or no speech to make themselves heard – they might not be used to being asked.

When there's a specific performance goal and an agreed rehearsal schedule, stick to it. If people are serious about becoming musicians it's important that they experience how much hard work and repetition is involved in getting it right and doing it well.

The toughest 'stick or shift' decision is probably when the room is divided: when some people are getting a lot out of what's happening and some are not. Activities won't please all of the people all of the time. Varying content, in terms of learning-style and musical content, increases the chances that people will find something to engage with. It helps to be well-staffed with people who can support participation and sometimes take people off to do something else if the session is really not working for them. Reviewing sessions (see the stories that follow each Activity Plan in Chapter 11) is a useful means of considering any issues regarding group mix and the most productive content for future sessions.

Large Music Group Session Plans

The template I use to plan a session always looks like this.

It gives me a space to:

- list the resources I need to prepare or take with me to the session
- write out a structured plan
- write ideas, observations and reflections during the session or straight after the session.

Activity Plan: Venue: Date: Time: Activity Session:	
Aims:	
Resources:	
Time:	Activity:
Review and ideas for the future:	

Sample plans

This chapter goes through 11 session plans and lists some other session ideas. The session plans described have been used in different places and with different people. Some are groups and some are workshop sessions, so they vary in duration.

The plans demonstrate how to use the template and how to structure a plan. I write down whatever helps me to plan, structure and reflect... I don't always complete all the boxes and never do it just for the sake of it. After each plan there is a piece of reflective writing. These give some background about where ideas came from, explain some of the things described in the plan including the equipment used, describe the ideas for further sessions that were generated in the session and identify some of the things that worked well.

Sample Activity Plan 1

Activity Plan:	
Venue: **Time:**	**Date:**
Activity Session: A trip to the moon	
Aims: In this session we will: Create and explore a multi-sensory, outer space environment Experiment with movement – moon walking Do some listening Think about how music paints scenes/pictures Work on instrumental and conducting skills Have fun	
Resources: Black-out curtains with glow in the dark stars, lava lamps and optic fibre lights from the sensory room. Digital recorder, amplifier, instruments. Space CDs. *Music Express* photocopiables.	

Time:	Activity:
	Set up room with chairs in close circle in the centre. Chairs will be the rocket, outside will be space.
5 mins	**Ice breakers**: Free dance to CDs – Walking on the Moon
	Lift off: Count down with the theme from Thunderbirds and Makaton signs to throw a ball, launch balloons off the parachute, jump.
10 mins	1. **Song**: Sing and play along to Space Oddity on CD – loud. Split into two groups – one to do count down. Use instrumental break for percussion jam. Turn out room lights, pull curtains so we can see glow stars and turn on optic fibre lights, climb into the rocket.

cont.

15 mins	2. **Listen to soundscape**: use Vangelis and Moonscape from *Music Express* 6 to listen to space sounds.
10/15 mins	**Comfort break**
20 mins	3. **Compose a space soundscape**. Play segment of Soundscape again; talk about why it sounds like space – agree the sets of sounds we need.
	• Split into groups to find sets of sounds needed for space soundscape. Each group to prepare a rhythm or riff.
	• Each group to play to each other.
	• Try mixing sounds from the groups – try some conducting.
	• Make a digital recording.
	• Play back through amplifier with lights out and space lighting on again.
8 mins	**Cool down**: leave lights down – CD Arvo Pärt, fade to silence. Leave lights down for a few minutes before moving.
Review and ideas for the future: Use moon landing film (*Music Express*) as silent movie to score. Make space soundscape into graphic score that looks like space. Do – Songs I would send into space to introduce me to an alien (and tell the story of Voyager – with listening time for some of the tracks that went on it).	

The story of the trip to the moon session

I arrived early to set up the room before the group arrived. It was well worth doing that; they walked into a space environment that was different from the group room they were used to and they were curious about it.

The count downs and blasting off were a big success.

I had one astronaut helmet with a mic in it – it would have been nice if we'd had one each.

Space Oddity was great with loud surround sound. It's a lovely, atmospheric piece of music to sing, dance and move to.

The Vangelis piece is quite eerie and I'd wondered if it might be a bit unsettling, but the group were quick to identify the features that made it sound like space.

The glow stars didn't work as well as I'd hoped, it just wasn't dark enough but the lights and blackout were really effective.

The group really got into the composition. The photocopiables in *Music Express 5* (Hanke 2003a) were useful for helping people identify types of sound they wanted. (*Music Express* are a set of teaching resource books with CDs and copiable.)

Group work – some of the activities were fairly solitary; some were co-operative. I could have included these factors as aims – but they were incidental to the musical activities rather than what drove them.

We often end with relaxation, listening and quiet time. We often end quietly so that people can re-enter the world a little calmly, because for some people the stopping is the hard bit.

What happened next?

I'd read a piece in *Music!* (DeGraffenreid *et al.* 2006) about Voyager and the tracks that were recorded and put on it so that the human race could introduce itself to Aliens. At the end of this moon session I gave out blank introduction cards (Hello Alien, I'm… and I'd like you to hear some of my favourite music). Each group member took one away, filled it in and brought their tracks to the next group. We travelled to the moon again (where an alien was waiting to meet us) I introduced them to some of the tracks that were on Voyager (from Beethoven's 5th, to Bach, some world music and Chuck Berry's Johnny Be Good). Then they each introduced and played their tracks and said as little or as much about them as they liked. It was a really nice way of introducing them to some classical pieces and also for them to share some of their own choices with the rest of the group.

We didn't make a graphic score of our moonscape, but it certainly would have lent itself to that.

Sample Activity Plan 2

Activity Plan:
Venue: Date:
Time:
Activity Session: Jack and the sound effect – story telling
Aims: In this session we will: Explore the use of sound as metaphor Listen actively to a story to identify where we could add sound effects Think about character, story and meaning Work on a performance Use rhythm to think about rhyming words (as a precursor to writing song lyrics)

cont.

Resources: props, story in rhyme, laminated symbols, magic chicken, chocolate eggs, the cymbala. Instruments and everyday objects for sound effects. Voice changer.

Time:	Activity:
5 mins	**Ice breaker**: Animal Fair – feet stamping to keep beat, sound effects, and ostinato (Monkey Monkey). All together and then divide into groups.
5 mins	**Set the scene and guess the story**: A casket (an old jewellery box) with clues inside it (objects of reference) – gold coins, coloured dried beans, leaves from a plant, a golden egg.
15 mins	**Story telling and sound effects**: Talk about the story and decide what sound effects you need – a growing bean stalk, a cow, climbing, a stomping giant, a snoring giant, a magic harp, a chicken, the tinkling of gold coins, chopping with an axe, the crash of the falling bean stalk, etc. Split into groups to find specific sound effects.
15 mins	**Use of voice**: Demonstrate the voice changing megaphone. Pass around so everyone can have a go. Choose a voice for our giant. Practise Fee Fi Foe Fumming! Demo the magic chicken and get it to lay some golden chocolate eggs for our tea break.
10/15 mins	**Tea and comfort break**
10 mins	Each group to demo the sound effects they've worked out.
20 mins	**The story**: Two story tellers, one to read the story (it's in rhyme) and one to hold up symbol cards when we need a sound effect. Loads of sound effects and audience participation.
5 mins	**Cool down**: Sleeping giants – snoring, then silent – listen to the sounds in the room.

Review and ideas for the future: music that tells a story – *Peter and the Wolf*.

Set up some one-to-one time with the people that enjoyed the cymbala.

The story of Jack and the sound effect story telling

Stories are part of how we pass on our culture. In cultures with low literacy rates (both historically and today) oral story telling is strong. Aside from the fact that it's a really nice, gentle, sharing social thing to do stories have all sorts of other relevance.

Every other year there's an International Disability Studies Conference in Lancaster – the focus is very much on the Social Model of Disability. In 2010 there was a workshop session about story telling. The speakers were people who told or collected stories across a range of cultures and used them to explore disability issues. One speaker talked of the value in encouraging disabled people to talk about which characters in a story they identified with and to use story as a means of conveying their own messages. One told *The Changeling* story and suggested this reflected the deep-seated belief in many cultures that impairment was a punishment. It got me thinking about the dying art of story telling in our culture and about how valuable it is, perhaps particularly if you are not literate, as a means of conveying personal messages about how we see ourselves and what we want to say.

We have used stories in group sessions several times. When we do, I try to find rhyming versions (it's usually easy thanks to the internet). Rhyme is a useful tool to explore speech patterns both for lyric writing and for encouraging speech (I expect there's some evidence that supports this opinion – I don't know of it – I just do it because it makes sense and it works). The speech rhythms of any culture are reflected in their musical rhythms (see Music and language in Chapter 2) and so it makes sense to explore rhyme as a precursor to musical rhythm too.

Stories we've used to make sound effects include *Jack and the Beanstalk, The Three Little Pigs, Goldilocks and the Three Bears* and *The Owl and the Pussy Cat.* The fairy tales are particularly good because of the well-known and repeated phrases they contain. People will often just recite them automatically (Fee, Fi, Fo Fum; I'll Huff and I'll Puff; Who's Been Sleeping in my Bed?, etc.).

As a next step, in exploring the relationship between lyrics and melody, I use poetry-reading over instrumental music (I read – *The Night Before Christmas* – over a track from The Musical Advent Calendar, as our cool down for a pre-Christmas session).

The Magic Harp is a cymbala; a flat sound box strung like a harp. It has coded music on cards that slide between the sound box and the strings. The melodies are played by plucking the strings over the coded pattern, like tracing an outline. It makes a lovely sound and is a useful way of getting people to understand rising and falling pitches and to read simple notation. Some of the people in the group really liked it and I did some one-to-one and a small group session with those who wanted to try playing the melodies. We went on to use it to compose; drawing our own patterns on card (a bit like a graphic score) and then putting them under the strings to play their shape and see what they sounded like.

The Magic Chicken is a home-made papier mâché sculpture; it has an internal sloping tunnel so that I can get it to lay magic eggs on request. We use it at Easter too, to convert Easter egg hunt bounty into chocolate. It's just a multi-sensory prop...but a little magic goes a long way!

The voice changer is a megaphone that has ten different voice changing settings. It's a great way of experimenting with voice and also of making yourself really loud. For the story it was used by the giant. We've used it on a couple of songs, first as a Maroon 5 tribute (She Will be Loved has synthesised vocals) and also in response to the immortal REM line 'A public service announcement followed me home the other day' which we used as inspiration for our song 'It's Been a Good Day' (see Appendix 1).

I use sound effects as a step towards abstract music that either tells stories or paints pictures. Some of the sound effects in Jack and the Beanstalk are literal – like the harp playing, others are about metaphor – a growing beanstalk. Developing ideas about these kinds of sound is essential to both understanding and composing instrumental works.

Stories have provided the inspiration for many classical works. We've used Prokofiev's Peter and the Wolf as an accessible way to follow what happens when you ascribe instrument and theme to various characters, because the story is told as it's played. Richard Strauss's Til Eulenspiegel is another example of how music can be used to also tell a story, without using words.

The Kalevala (Mäkinen 2009) is the book of Finnish folklore and was often inspiration for Sibelius. It's also inspired much art and poetry so it's a rich vein for project work. I have a beautiful translation with lots of coloured illustrations and have used it to introduce the group to Sibelius.

Ballet works (Swan Lake, The Nut Cracker, Romeo and Juliet) are useful too since the connection between the story and the music are concrete, particularly if you have DVD or can go to a performance of the ballet rather than just listen to the music.

Silence is a valuable commodity. I never use it for long, but I do use it quite often. I think sometimes in our eagerness to give people activity the world becomes too frenetic a place and can be incredibly disabling for people who are hyper-sensitive or who struggle to screen out white noise. I've been very struck by one or two of the people I have worked with who respond very positively to silence (see Shane's journey, Chapter 9).

Sample Activity Plan 3

Activity Plan:	
Venue:	**Date:**
Time:	
Activity Session: Pictures at an Exhibition, Session 1 (Project to run over several sessions)	

Aims: In this session we will:
Understand and follow the form of a large-scale piece of classical music
Explore how music paints pictures and pictures can inspire music
Compose and perform our own piece that has the same form as Pictures at an Exhibition
Produce a musical product that can be performed in public without live performance

Resources:
Expression cards. Pictures. Range of art, craft media for painting, collage, etc. Digital recorder. Recording of Mussorgsky's Pictures at an Exhibition.

Time:	Activity:
10 mins	**Ice breaker**: Musical Expressions – walk around the room to the promenade music. When the music stops make a face (laminated cards, call them out and use Makaton signs) Happy, Sad, Bored, Angry, Shy, Surprised, Frightened, Excited.
10 mins	**Talk about going to a gallery or seeing an art exhibition**: Who has done that? What do you do? Then play samples of the promenade music in its different arrangements – Can people hear it's the same tune? Can they sing it?
20 mins	**Introduce the form of Pictures at an Exhibition**: Explain that we are going to write our own piece that's this shape too.
	Play extracts from the piece alternating Promenade with Pictures – ask people to guess what the pictures are.
	Over three sessions:
	1. Compose our own Promenade: think about pulse and tempo. (Use dice for melody against speech rhythm of a song.)

cont.

2. Split into groups: Select pictures from a choice cut from magazines photos, etc. – each group to choose one picture and compose a soundscape to represent it.

3. Each group to paint a picture that reflects their soundscape.

4. Pictures up on the wall. All to play Promenade and then groups to take turns to play their picture – returning to promenade each time. Record the piece.

5. Make frames for pictures. Put on an exhibition with our piece running on a loop.

Cool down: Don McLean's Vincent with Van Gogh PowerPoint.

Review and ideas for the future: Painting to pieces of music – paint sample squares and build a big musical mosaic. Use puppets to explore expressions.

The story of the Pictures at an Exhibition project

Some of the people in the group have difficulty interpreting facial expressions which leads to an inability to make ones that other people understand too. The ice breaker is one I repeat intermittently to give them an opportunity to try out their own expressions and to see other people's in response to specific mood words, signs and symbols. We like this ice breaker – everyone really hams it up, it's very funny. It's a confidence building/drama activity but I like also to make the connections about code; spoken language, facial expression, pictures and music are all forms of code that are open to interpretation.

Most of the group had never been to an exhibition so we described one and acted it out. Some of the people in the group get very anxious about trying new things so I hope our exhibition will, in part, be a rehearsal for a trip to a museum or gallery.

The project gave us lots of things to work on:

- The simple ABA'CA''D form of the Mussorgsky (where A is the promenade theme which recurs, slightly changed but very recognisable, between each picture – the pictures are B, C, etc.) was easy to follow and to mirror in our own composition.

- The promenade in the Mussorgsky is in 2/2 time. It conveys the beat produced by walking. We used the idea of composing in 2/2 so we could walk to it.

Our promenade music was composed using the dice method (see Chapter 8). I wondered how to give the melody an interesting rhythm. We meet, and some of the group members live in a house surrounded by countryside. The guys often go on long country walks and sometimes sing with their support workers whilst they're walking. The Wheels on the Bus is a favourite walking song for one of our group members; she often doesn't speak and she finds it difficult to concentrate for long, but this song will usually get her joining in – so we borrowed the rhythm and put our dice melody against it.

- Interpreting music. First we guessed what the 'pictures' in the Mussorgsky were, describing or painting the scene they evoked for each of us. Then we created a whole set of pictures of our own.

I prepared a big pile of laminated pictures so that the group could choose the pictures that would inspire our cameos. The ones they chose were a tiger in a river, a rocket on a launch pad, a starry sky, a castle by a lake, a close-up of a pile of coloured glass marbles.

We worked in small groups to produce short fragments of music – one inspired by each picture. Then we used the fragments to inspire a whole new set of our own paintings, drawings, collages, sculptures and masks (we used different materials for each fragment so that the art work was very varied). We worked with the art tutor in a joined-up project that resulted in a large scale and very concrete product: a gallery of paintings that could be grouped in families of very different works and set out as an art exhibition with our own original music as a backdrop.

The music is digitally recorded. I'm hoping we will get to put on an exhibition where the pictures are displayed, as at an art exhibition, and the music runs on a loop. Some of the group find the idea of live performance completely terrifying, others get very distracted by the setting and then can't concentrate to perform live. Music is often 'in the moment' and it can be much more difficult to produce an end-product than when working with a different medium (like cooking or gardening). This project gave us an exhibition derived from our music work: a performance/installation piece where people could exhibit what they'd achieved in a real time way without the pressure of live performance.

For the cool down, the Van Gogh PowerPoint was downloaded from the internet and shown on multi-media projector (MMP). It's a slide show of Van Gogh paintings that roll over Don McLean's Vincent – it's beautiful: poignant, moving and calming and a perfect illustration of the connection between visual and musical code and how these can be used together to convey a message.

Using puppets

One of the faces someone made during the ice breaker reminded me of the sock puppets I'd made as a child. We made sock puppets at a future session; everyone had their own, they looked very different (hair styles, glasses, eyes, etc.). We used them first to play with expressions (I even found a page of sock puppet expressions on the internet for us to try and copy). Then we set up a stage and the guys each puppet-danced or sang to a favourite track. It's a good way of getting people on stage and performing without them having to put themselves physically there: no one could see them, they could use their own voices or play with different ones, but it was their character that was there and it was them that was deciding how it played out. We filmed it so they could watch themselves afterwards.

Sample Activity Plan 4

Activity Plan:	
Venue:	Date:
Time:	
Activity Session: Song writing	
Aims: In this session we will: Take apart and then perform The Lazy Song (Bruno Mars) Look at the film for and listen to The JCB Song (Nizlopi) Talk about the things that make these songs work Start writing our own song inspired by these two	
Resources: Multi-media projector and lap top	

Time:	Activity:
10 mins	**Ice breaker**: Dance, sing and play along to The Lazy Song.
40 mins	**Activity**: Split into groups: percussion, drums, chords (guitar, glock and keyboard). Listen to the song again focusing on the role your instrument plays. Give out composition block score to each group. Each group to rehearse separately.
10 mins	Put it back together and perform the song. **Tea break (and set up MMP)**

40 mins	Run JCB song with animation, through MMP.
	Turn the sound off and run again – singing to guitar. Talk about the bits we like and what makes it work (4/4, major key, simple melody, childlike story telling, etc.).
	Choose chord palette for our own composition. Tell some childhood memory stories and use these to generate lyrics.
	Rerun both tracks to end.

Review and ideas for the future:

The song writing session story

Breaking down a favourite song and making it playable is often really straightforward. You're most likely to need some drums, some percussion (tambourine, wood blocks, shakers), something to play chords on (guitar, uke, keyboard) and singing.

Most popular songs are written in 4/4 (four whole beats to a bar). In 4/4 the first beat of the bar is usually the most important – clap along to the song, make the first of each four beats louder – if this fits then the chances are it's in 4/4.

Split the group into small groups. Ask one group to keep a steady four beats to a bar either by clapping, stamping feet or playing drums. Emphasise the first beat by asking another group just to play that (perhaps on a different type of drum). The second most important beat in 4/4 is often the third beat of the bar – ask one group to play tambourines on the first and third beat… that's drums and percussion sorted. The same pattern will work for a huge number of pop songs.

Any piece of music, that doesn't have significant key changes, can be harmonised with just three chords (the original may or may not be more complicated but three chords will work). For chord players mark up chords with colour-coded stickers (see 'Enabling Participation in Music' (Chapter 8)) and open-tune stringed instruments. For those playing strings who don't finger chords – The Lazy Song works perfectly well with an instrument open-tuned in D and played throughout (it sounds really good with an open-tuned ukulele (see Appendix 2) playing over picked guitar chords).

I use composition blocks as simple scores to help people remember what they're doing (see Appendix 3).

Nizlopi's JCB song was a big favourite with one group member, so he brought it for us to hear. It's a great song and the animation that goes with it is lovely. There are a couple of things about it that I felt made it particularly relevant: it's childlike, not childish and the sound has an innocence and purity that modern pop doesn't provide very often and the lyrics too are a refreshing departure from the usual mainstream. The group provide the lyrics for the songs we write. They are very much about their experience of the world: none of them have girl or boyfriends, none of them drive cars or have jobs. A song like this is a validation, I think, of the powerful effect of writing about what you know, what you understand about your world. So we used the JCB song as the starting point for some personal story swapping – memories of childhood, stories from school. All of the ideas in the lyrics of Scaletrix and Stickle Bricks have been spun from the stories we told each other.

Scaletrix and Stickle Bricks was the title track of our first, home-produced CD – Gavin drew the CD cover which makes reference in both style and content to the JCB song animation, and it is on the cover of this book.

Sample Activity Plan 5

Activity Plan: Venue: Date: Time: Activity Session: Cake baking, cake form composition and graphic scoring (2 sessions on same day)	
Aims: In this session we will: Develop a compositional idea by using an everyday process Develop skills in making and performing from a graph score Have a good time…and eat cake	
Resources: Flip chart and pens, cake making ingredients.	
Time:	**Activity:**
10 mins	**Ice breaker**: Favourite cake percussion. Make a list of favourite cakes. Try them all out, and then try cross rhythms (Victoria sandwich, double chocolate muffin, carrot cake…).
5 mins	**Set up session**: Explain that we're going to write a piece of instrumental music that has the same shape as making a cake.

25 mins	**Cake making**: Make a list, as you go, of the process (creaming, beating, folding) and the ingredients. Whilst it's cooking and cooling…
40 mins	**Composition**: Select instruments and how they will be played at each stage: Draw as a rough score, chose a conductor, perform and record.
	Decorate cake. Eat cake, drink tea and have a break.
20 mins	**Set up art stuff and a large single sheet for the score:** Paint, draw, and collage cake form graphic score. Choose how each instrument (ingredient) will be represented and when it will appear.

Review and ideas for the future:
Think of other everyday processes and use them to inspire composition.

Story of the cake score session

I wanted a way of exploring form, in music, that would make sense to people. It occurred to me one day when I was cooking tea that preparing food usually has a step-wise process that is made up of different tasks. Cake making actually has a very musical shape (it's not so very far removed from sonata-form); and it's something that either people have done or, on the whole, they're very happy to try doing.

Food is great for making sessions multi-sensory: it adds taste, smell, colour and touch immediately. I tend to only include food occasionally because I think it's nice for it to be unexpected, but I do include it either as described here (to help explain something) or as a means of contributing to scene setting (see Activity Plans 6 and 8).

There are lots of ways that everyday processes can be used to reflect or inspire musical form: a car journey, a day out, having a bath, building a house, having a conversation with a friend, etc..

Many classical pieces are written in the shape of a story or a day out with each movement setting a different scene: Picnic on the Marne and Tableaux de Provence are two pieces in the classical sax repertoire that do the latter.

I once watched the Mike Westbrook band play a piece they called Trifle: movement by movement a different instrument took the lead and they built a trifle from the bottom up (sponge, jelly, custard, cream, sprinkles).

I remember too, once hearing of a contemporary composer who had written a piece based on working through the levels of a computer platform game – working through the levels with the same little recurring character riff returning throughout.

Anything in day-to-day life can be taken to inspire musical form and having that form in mind gives the composition a shape, a character an ebb and flow that makes it sound much more accomplished than an unstructured piece.

A process also lends itself beautifully to graphic scoring, and if you use attractive materials scores can be very artistic. Our cake-making score was on a long sheet of black card and we used metallic stars, glitter pens and collage to build a score that read from left to write across the page and ended up looking like a beautiful swirling galaxy; it looked nothing like a cake or cake making, it just had the same underlying process. We could have made the connection more concrete, but it didn't feel necessary and I think it was valuable to demonstrate that we could do something abstract and because we knew how we got there, go back to it later and read it like a map.

Sample Activity Plan 6

Activity Plan:	
Venue:	**Date:**
Time:	
Activity Session: Chinese New Year	
Aims: In this session we will: Mark Chinese New Year Listen to some traditional Chinese music Begin to compose a song inspired by traditional Chinese music Make a Chinese dancing dragon Practise dancing together including leading and following and being very close to each other	
Resources: Scrap cardboard, PVA, kitchen roll, paint and length of material for dragon. Pictures. CDs of traditional Chinese music. Fortune cookies. Sop sax and Chinese folk sheet music. Fortune cookies. Instrument box – including hanging chimes, bells, Chinese symbols, wooden xylophone.	

Time:	Activity:
10 mins	**Ice breaker:** Chinese New Year animals. Use Chinese calendar to tell individuals the animal of their birth year. Each person to act as their animal – movement, sounds, etc. and to try to identify the other people in the group with the same animal.

40 mins	**Project:** Look at Chinese dragon dancing pictures, then start building our own Chinese dragon.
	Practise walking and then dancing to Chinese music in a line – leader and follower, staying together, touching each other. Try to move on to doing this under the fabric that will be the dragon's tail.
10 mins	**Tea and fortune cookies**
30 mins	**Song writing:** Read out fortune cookie proverbs and pick out our favourite ones. Talk about what we like about them, what they make us think of – write ideas down on flip chart as we go so we can use these as a basis for lyrics for a Chinese New Year inspired song.
	Listening to Chinese folk melodies: First on CD. Then live performance. Talk about how they sound, picking out and demonstrating the things about rhythm, mode and instrumentation that create a traditional Chinese sound.
10 mins	Choose the features and instruments we will use to write our own Chinese inspired music.
	Work out what we need to do next time: End with Chinese meditation music for relaxation.

Review and ideas for the future: Do something with people's Chinese animals…

The Chinese New Year Story

Chinese New Year celebrations are colourful, vibrant and alive with Chinese music and dance; a perfect combination for some multi-sensory project work and a good opportunity to explore a sound palette that is easy to engage with but is very different from our western European one.

The Chinese dragon worked out well. It is made of cardboard boxes, toilet rolls and egg boxes – coated in kitchen roll and PVA and painted in hot colours. He took a few sessions to complete and is like a huge team puppet.

Dancing the dragon is not only a real team effort, it also means that people have to be very close together: both are things that aren't easy for many of the people in the group, but they are made much more possible when the focus is on a task (dancing the dragon) rather than the actions it takes to achieve it.

The fortune cookies worked well: they added a sensory dimension (taste) and were a food no one in the group had ever tried. Each contained a Chinese proverb: Chinese philosophy is warm and gentle and positive. The proverbs gave plenty to talk about and some nice material for song lyrics.

Chinese music isn't entirely alien; people have heard it on films and computer games, and some of the people in the group also do Tai Chi together. It has enough in common with the music we're used to that it is easy music to listen to, but it is also markedly different in some respects. Thinking about that difference (in terms of rhythm, timbre and key) and then trying to create something that used those features provided us with lots of learning.

The Chinese animals inspired a totem pole sculpture and the Chinese dragon held centre-stage for a procession and is safely stored away to use again.

Sample Activity Plan 7

Activity Plan:	
Venue:	Date:
Time:	
Activity Session: Halloween	

Aims: In this session we will:
Jump the broomstick
Use magic spells to develop percussion rhythms and song lyrics
Think up and try some spooky sound effects
Look at the relationship between film and music
Work on conducting and following a conductor as a performer

Resources: Broomsticks and wands, spells and magic charms – with picture cards, sound effect spooky story – with picture cards, multimedia projector, Fantasia.

Time:	Activity:
15 mins	**Ice breaker**: Jump the broomstick
40 mins	**Activity**:
	• Read spells and charms aloud.
	• Work in groups to develop sound effects to go with each.
	• Demonstrate an underlying percussive pulse (ostinato) and how we can use it to keep the piece moving forward and make it coherent.
	• Set up the ostinato and each group to perform their section in turn to form a whole piece.
	Tea break (set up MMP)

10 mins	Use picture cards to agree sound effects.
20 mins	Spontaneous performance: one person to read spooky story, one to conduct (hold up the appropriate picture cards) for the rest of the group to perform.
20 mins	Fantasia – Night on a Bare Mountain (as example of story with music).
10 mins	**Cool down:** Try conducting with Leopolski and Mickey Mouse.
Review and ideas for the future:	

The Halloween story

Dance is a natural way to encourage fluid movement and dancing with or around an object adds interest and challenge. We Jumped the Broomsticks, made arches with them to dance under and through, we rode them, we raced them.

The broomsticks and the wands were home-made – from hazel and willow, tied with lovely natural twine, plaited with coloured ribbons, sprayed with multi-coloured glitter: they were beautiful sensory objects of reference, there to be enjoyed.

Spells and chants have a rhythmic energy so they're great to play to. Creating a 'song' from them can be fairly simple. A melody isn't essential; a soundscape can be created using spell sound effects. Use really short effects and just keep repeating them as if they're on a loop (or record them and generate a loop), then speak your spells or chants over the top. Experiment with horror voices, try a voice changer.

Fantasia is a classic film and this was a good opportunity to use it to look at the relationship between music and picture. It's unusual in that the animation was designed to reflect the music rather than visa versa. It's also a really positive way to introduce some wonderful classical music.

Conducting and being conducted is a useful way of experiencing many musical and non-musical things (see Chapter 8, 'Enabling Participation in Music').

Standing in front of the MMP allowed us to create shadow conductors on the screen and to conduct with Leopolski and Mickey Mouse, just for fun.

Sample Activity Plan 8

Activity Plan:	
Venue:	Date:
Time:	
Activity Session: Bonfire Night sensory session	

Aims: Bright, colourful, fun multi-sensory session
Activities free-flowing and taking as much or as little time as seems useful
Orientation and a bit of story-telling
An accessible fireworks display – where we can manage noise levels

Resources: Material to fake a bonfire...apples on sticks, chocolate, etc., MMP, DVD.

Time:	Activity:
10 mins	**Ice breaker:** Parachute with ribbons and balloons.
20 mins	**Chocolate apples and marsh mallows:** Melt chocolate and dip apples and marsh mallows on sticks, then roll in chocolate sprinkles, and leave to set.
20 mins	**Campfire songs:** Build an indoor campfire (outdoors if it's nice) and sing campfire songs – Campfire's Burning, Oh You'll Never go to Heaven, Ging Gang Gooley, Do Your Ears Hang Low, etc.
15 mins	**Comfort and tea break:** Drinking chocolate too. And eat the food we've just made.
20 mins	**Firework display:** DVD with classic rock soundtrack on multi-media projector. Lights down.
10 mins	Tell the Guy Fawkes story with shadow puppets on MMP screen.
10 mins	Finish with DVD fireworks on silent.

Review and ideas for the future: Puppets and shadow puppets, using self as shadow – Me and My Shadow.

Story of the Bonfire Night session

Some of the people in the group are very frightened by unpredictable sound – I wanted them to experience an enjoyable firework display. The ice breaker mimics some of the things that are nice about fireworks. The ribbons are in streamers with a bound end – so they can be thrown up and spread out as they fall. We used them and a big pile of chiffon pieces of different rainbow colours and launched them off the parachute by rippling it. The balloons, are long thin ones, again multi-coloured. We blew them up and let them go, they shot around the room and whistle…a bit like fireworks (not everyone liked them).

It sometimes surprises me the kind of music that the people in the group know, but the campfire songs were chosen because I was fairly confident that two of the people in the group who speak infrequently, would know and sing them – they did. We built a bonfire (it was pouring with rain so it was a fake one I'm afraid – a pile of sticks and logs over a light) and sang loads of cheesy campfire songs – with actions, as rounds, etc. – they were a big hit.

Toffee apples are one of my own firework night memories…but I've always thought they look so much nicer than they taste and also melted toffee is so hot it would have limited how it could be used and who by…so we melted white and milk chocolate and used it for dipping apples and marsh mallows. They were very delicious and we'll definitely be looking for reasons to do it again! It wasn't essential to the music, obviously, but it was fun and it helped evoke the atmosphere. I don't feel any pressure for the sessions I facilitate to be entirely music focused. Music runs through what we do; sometimes it's absolutely central, sometimes it's just there as part of what's happening, sometimes we stop the music altogether because something else has become more important – and that something else may or may not have been elicited by the music.

I love using the multi-media projector (MMP). As long as the room's big enough we can make the screen huge against a neutral coloured wall. It produces a muted image that's not too overwhelming. It worked well with the fireworks – we had them all over the room, walls and ceiling, just by playing a DVD of a rather grand display. The DVD gave a choice of soundtracks – original, classical, classic rock – the group chose the rock. I showed them a bit of the classical too because I love the way that whatever music you play against any film it not only looks like it's meant to be there, but it changes the character of the visual image. The display is also really lovely on silent so we used that too, as our cool down.

I saw a display once where the bonfire was a mock-up of the Houses of Parliament and giant actors with stilts and papier mâché heads acted out the alternative Guy Fawkes story (where he succeeded in blowing up the House – the stage was set alight and the fireworks all went off at once at the end of the story); it was engaging and impressive. One of the group read a rhyming version of the Guy Fawkes story whilst some of the others did a shadow puppet performance against the backdrop of the fireworks display: it provided a story telling opportunity, with a little performance practice built in too.

Some of the group really like the multi-media projector screen when there's nothing on it and they can see themselves as a shadow. We use it as a backdrop for dancing and we also use shadow puppets to achieve the same one step removed performance opportunity (see Activity Plan 3).

Sample Activity Plan 9

Activity Plan:	
Venue: Date:	
Time:	
Activity Session: Focusing on use of voice	

Aims: In this session we will:
Encourage everyone to use their voice
Play with vocal sounds that rely upon made up words (Scat)
Think about increasing voice projection and volume without vocal strain
Encourage speech through song
Make a lot of noise.

Resources: CDs, mic, guitar, etc.

Time:	Activity:
10 mins	**Ice breaker:** Hat and mic.
10 mins	**Voice training exercises:** Focus on posture, diaphragm support, projection and volume.
15 mins	**Voice sounds to CD:** Prince Charming, Who Let the Dogs Out? Mahna Mahna.
15 mins	**Songs with vocal sound effects:** With guitar How Much is that Doggie?, Old MacDonald, The Runaway Train.
15 mins	**Songs with sentence finishing or echo:** Do Wah Diddy Diddy, Mony Mony, Shout, Crocodile Rock, Big Yellow Taxi, Walking on Sunshine.
15 mins	**Comfort break**
20 mins	**Play some Scat on CD whilst drinking tea:** Ella Fitzgerald, Blues Brothers. Try Sing Scat from *Music Express*. Do Mini the Moocher, with guitar – lead first then try volunteers, use mic!
10 mins	**Cool down:** Sirening to parachute until it's so low we can't hear it, then silence.
Review and ideas for the future:	

Story of the vocal session

From time to time we do sessions with no musical instruments (or perhaps just my guitar) and focus solely on the sounds people make. Whilst many of the people in the group have little or no speech they all use their voices sometimes. These sessions are to give time and space to experiment with voice, to encourage those who use it quietly and infrequently to use it and expect to be heard, to encourage those who have some words to speak, to encourage those who speak and sing to use their voices carefully (see Gavin's journey in Chapter 9).

Hat and mic

We use lots of variations of this ice breaker, but basically we pass round a cool hat and a microphone to music and when it stops…the person with the mic introduces the person with the hat in some way and the person in the hat has a bit of solo time if they want it.

Voice training exercises

I dip in and out of Mike Brewer's *Warm Ups!* (2002) and use the exercises he sets out to introduce some ideas and try them out. It's easier to engage people if it's fun (we like the sirening and the pretending to be a monkey exercises!). It's also a useful way of focusing on posture; many of the people in the group, for a wide range of reasons, don't naturally sit or stand actively, rather they lean on their skeletons or on their chair and many prefer to look at the floor than to look up: we can use vocalising to see what happens if you change your posture. We use the diaphragm support, projection and volume exercises and when we're as loud as we think we can be we try one, two, three – shout (whatever you like) and see who hears who…then, when we're good and noisy we try our voices against song CD tracks that use vocal sound (rather than speech) to create their mood.

Voice sounds to CD

Try Prince Charming (Adam and the Ants), Who Let the Dogs Out? (Baha Men), Mahna Mahna (The Muppets). Some of these songs, especially the Adam and the Ants tracks, are quite primal and, if you really let go, very energising to vocalise with – we really enjoy it! We've also used CDs of Native American chants.

Songs with vocal sound effects – with guitar

For some reason (the logic of which escapes me) people as children, whether they have speech or not are taught to make animal noises (what does the doggy say?). It's a starting point, in terms of vocalising, that people often relate to and so I use it as that – a place to start and to move on from (see Age appropriateness in Chapter 7). We use songs like How Much is That Doggie?, Old MacDonald and The Runaway Train with Makaton signs and laminated symbols.

Songs with sentence finishing or echo

I think of this as a developmental approach (see Chapter 5). The next step on from vocal sounds is sentence finishing. People often finish each other's sentences in everyday conversation; it's very natural and it also makes use of the positive reinforcement people get from completing things (see backward chaining in 'The OT Tool Kit', Chapter 5).

The songs we use (e.g. Do Wah Diddy Diddy, Mony Mony, Shout, Crocodile Rock, Big Yellow Taxi, Walking on Sunshine) are, on the whole, loud, driving, feel-good songs that are hard to resist and either have short vocal riffs in the choruses, vocal breaks or places where a backing group echo back what the soloist sings.

There's a whole tradition of Scat singing – perhaps best known courtesy of Ella Fitzgerald, the Rat Pack and Cleo Lane. Scat is ideal because having sounds but not words is a positive advantage! The people in the group who have speech tend to end up mimicking those who don't and trying out their sounds – which is great fun and is greatly enjoyed by one or two of the more vocal non-speakers!

Cool down

We use the visual cues from the parachute to bring people's voices slowly sirening back down, in both pitch and volume until it's so low we can't hear it. Sometimes we do it standing and I ask people to sit as their own voice stops or as they can't hear anyone else. We keep going until everyone has stopped and then just hold a few minutes silence: it's nice to feel the contrast…and being silent becomes altogether more attractive when you've also been loud and been heard.

Sample Activity Plan 10

Activity Plan:	
Venue:	Date:
Time:	
Activity Session: Sing a Rainbow	

Aims: In this session we will:
Create a tactile, colourful environment
Use a multi-sensory approach to teach/reinforce Makaton signs for colours
Sing and play and dance some songs
Have solo time, instrument and improvising opportunities

Resources: Coloured chiffon scarves, Makaton sign book.

Time:	Activity:
20 mins	**Ice breaker**: Revise Makaton sign for 'Good Morning', play musical statues – greeting each other in the breaks.
10 mins	**Sing a Rainbow:** Each to choose scarf from the pile in the middle of the room. Go through colours – word, sign and scarf.
	Sing 'Sing a Rainbow' – signing colours and holding up scarf.
5 mins	**Set up activity for next two sessions:** To select a colour, see what songs we can think of that feature the colour, sing and play them, create a colour board of pictures, found objects, scarves and reference to the songs, for each colour.
	Today – Red, Orange, Yellow.
30 mins	**Scavenger hunt:** Small groups (one or two for each colour), take a scarf colour each and find objects of that colour, one for each descriptive word: shiny, soft, fluffy, round, square, perfumed, smooth, tickly, sticky.
10 mins	**Break (and set up colour tables)**

cont.

30 mins	**Songs:**
	Red: Lady in Red (solo sing with mic), Theme from Red Dwarf (jamming with instruments), Red Red Wine, 99 Red Balloons
	Orange: Oranges and Lemons (dance/action), Orange Crush
	Yellow: Yellow Submarine (ukes, drums, instrumental break), Tie a Yellow Ribbon (sing and decorate 'tree').
	Yellow: (singing with mic) – to end.

Review and ideas for the future:

The Sing a Rainbow story

I considered and avoided using Sing a Rainbow for years, it just seemed a bit…corny. It was an amazing session: several people in the group who rarely sing knew the song. I have a lovely recording of the whole group singing it. The scarves served as objects of reference and adding these to the signs gave people lots of cues.

The colour songs were all songs we'd used before, so were an opportunity to revisit and just enjoy the singing and playing.

I like scavenger hunts and we use them from time to time, as they are used here, to reinforce what we're doing by making the activities more diverse and by increasing the number of senses used (searching for, finding and carrying back objects is a multi-sensory activity).

Linking songs about colour and Makaton signs for colours to a table full of objects of that colour was a tangible way of demonstrating the concept of colours.

I made a 'tree' out of coppiced corkscrew hazel to use as the tree for Tie a Yellow Ribbon: again it was a song that people knew, attaching a concrete task to it illustrated the meaning of the words and also produced a beautiful sculpture.

We did the rest of the rainbow in the following session: Green Door, Blue Moon (lovely for harmonica breaks) and Purple Rain.

Sample Activity Plan 11

Activity Plan:	
Venue:	Date:
Time:	
Activity Session: Silent Movie Soundtrack	

Aims: In this session we will:
Explore the use of sound effects as simile and metaphor
See how sound is used for humour
Try some of our own sound effects
Look at how music is used to set scenes and create atmosphere on films

Resources: MMP and laptop, instruments, DVDS.

Time:	Activity:
20 mins	**Ice breaker:** Most interesting noise with an everyday object hunt.
20 mins	**Explore sound effects**
20 mins	**Watch short clip of silent film a few times.** Talk about what noises and try them.
	Rehearse and repeat.
10 mins	**Break**
10 mins	**Play** Rhapsody in Blue.
20 mins	Ben Britten's Night Mail with soundtrack and then with Gershwin.
20 mins	**Fantasia.**
10 mins	Arvo Pärts' Spiegal im Spiegal with DVD.

Review and ideas for the future:

The Silent Movie Soundtrack story

Creating sound effects to accompany silent film scenes is a good way of exploring the use of sound as simile and metaphor which in turn is a useful starting point in developing skills in understanding and interpreting music (see Chapter 8, 'Enabling Participation in Music').

The ice breaker is another variation on the scavenger hunt and encourages people to explore their environment – rustling plastic bags, opening and closing umbrellas, running drum sticks along radiators – all make great sound effects.

We explored the sounds by first hearing them and then picking pictures from a set of laminated cards and seeing which sounds worked with each picture.

The silent movie clip was Laurel and Hardy, a short scene involving all the usual slapstick moments: a kick up the rear, a falling object landing on someone's head and knocking them out, a ball being dropped at the top of and bouncing down a long staircase. We played randomly at first and then as the clip became more familiar the sound became more structured, specific effects were chosen for specific incidents and the incidents were then increasingly accurately anticipated and timed. We did this activity with very little talking, it just evolved by itself.

A steam train journey inspired Gershwin's Rhapsody in Blue...once you know that it's obvious. I wanted to see if any of the group could hear it without being told: several guesses were immediately close and with a short discussion one person did suggest it was a train. We listened to the sections where the musical representation of the pistons and the clacking of wheels on track can be clearly heard.

Night Mail is a black and white film that charts the overnight journey of a 1930s mail train. It sets a poem by W.H. Auden over music written by Benjamin Britten (specifically for the film) to great effect. We ran it once, then ran it again with Gershwin's Rhapsody in Blue playing and a third time with our own improvised soundtrack: I love the way that you can change the atmosphere of film very dramatically by changing the music.

Fantasia is a huge resource of soundtrack material – Mussorgsky's Night on a Bare Mountain is particularly atmospheric.

We often use a recording of Arvo Pärt's Spiegal im Spiegal as our cool down. YouTube has endless very effective versions of it being used as the soundtrack to films or series of photographs.

Some more ideas for sessions
Seasonal favourites

Calendar days and annual festivals are always inspiration for music-based activities because every important celebration in any culture has music at its heart (see Music as part of our everyday existence, p.22). We use celebrations to shape the passing year and also as an opportunity to explore cultures we're unfamiliar with. These can often be used as the subject of an ongoing project leading up to the celebration day. We mark the same ones and add a few more each year. When I first started to facilitate groups I felt that I had to come up with new ideas all of the time. Over the years what I've come to see is how nice it is sometimes to be utterly predictable! My Christmas at home is always the same – same routine, same meals, same music, same decorations in the same places, I love it like that and my now grown-up children would be less than pleased if I changed anything. So we've got a bit of a list of 'Let's do it like we did it last year' favourites.

Here are a few of them:

- **Beating the bounds:** A pagan ritual to wake up the trees at the beginning of Spring (adopted by the Christian Church to affirm the parish boundaries) and the perfect excuse to be outside playing very loud drums and decorating trees with wind chimes.

- **Maypole dancing:** We have a maypole that I've made out of junk yard scrap. It fits together like building a tower out of bricks – each of the group has decorated their own block with ribbons and mosaic. The top piece has all the long ribbons for dancing. We make up our own dances to folk CDs and dance outside if it's dry. Also a good excuse, once you've tangled up the maypole, for a bit of barn dancing and squeeze box playing.

- **Summer holidays:** Break out the summer favourites (Summer Holiday, The Beach Boys, Day Trip to Bangor) and the party dances (The Macarena, The Salsa, Oops Upside Your Head). Limbo dancing is great fun and really good to get people flexing and moving and bending (see Darren's journey in Chapter 9).

- **Advent:** A musical advent calendar with a different Christmas song or music for each day.

- **Christmas:** Carols and traditional songs obviously, but one of our favourite things is playing the handbells. We do it by colour and number with a big sheet of songs written out; each bell is a different colour and matched by its corresponding number. It takes a bit of preparing but it's well worth the effort.

CHAPTER 12

Small Group and One-to-One Sessions

The extent to which people's behaviour changes depending on the size of the group they're participating in is sometimes very striking. There's also a big difference between a large group in a large room and a large group in a smaller room. There isn't a blanket judgement to be made about which is better. What is important is that best use is made of each opportunity. Having the flexibility to work individually, in small groups and in larger groups gives everyone the best chance to work with their different selves and to focus on and experience different things. Accessibility is the central issue.

Types of engagement

People are all different. At any party they'll be those who take centre stage, those who get pleasure reacting to what is happening, those who like to watch it unfold and those who really aren't very comfortable being there. I'm circumspect about how I move the lime-light around in a large group; I tend, whilst making sure that people have enough support to do what they want to do, not to use activities that draw attention to people who seem very content just letting it all happen around them. For some people being immersed in the atmosphere without being the focus of attention is a very active choice and should be respected. It's critical that the value of experiences to individuals is judged by their own measure of that experience. When it's appropriate to encourage people who observe rather than actively participate or lead to experiment with and experience different roles, then it makes sense to do that first in a much smaller, quieter group.

Whatever the activity, a little individual attention makes you feel good and I think it's really worthwhile, if only because of that, to be able to work with people away from the big chaotic large group sometimes.

Small group sessions

Things work better in smaller groups when:

- listening and being able to hear yourself are important

- the task takes focus and concentration (e.g. song writing)

- experimenting with something new – a new role, a new skill (e.g. teaching instrument skills)

- working on a particular goal or interest that's shared with a few other people.

Sensory sessions

Large group sessions usually have multi-sensory elements but focused sensory sessions need to be small groups in order to make them successful. Specific sensory sessions are sometimes valuable for people who:

- are hypo- or hyper-sensitive to sensory stimulation

- are more likely to observe than actively participate in large groups

- are unable to join large group activities because of the noise level

- find sound quite frightening

- find movement frightening.

These sessions can be quite intense so are usually no more than half an hour in length. They work best when everyone has one-to-one support. They tend to be quiet, still spaces where silence is valued and sound is encouraged to just gently bubble up through it. We don't sing songs or experiment with instrumental riffs. We're much more likely to be sitting very quietly, in a circle, and using either just our bodies and our voices or using quiet hand-held percussion (bells, castanets) to make sound. I like establishing a silence and then giving a space for each person in turn to lead the sound that is made. Sometimes the group has far more silence than sound – and that can be the most important thing.

The secondary focus for the sensory sessions is often movement, particularly assisted movement, where the physical pressure of being held or moved increases the sensory feedback the individual experiences. Relaxing music (see Chapter 8, 'Enabling Participation in Music', relaxation music examples) or a recording of natural sound (rainfall or waves) can accompany:

- holding someone from behind, around their shoulders and gentle rocking

- gentle tapping of a pulse on someone's leg or shoulder

- swinging gently in the hammock

- gently bouncing someone sat on a fitness ball
- making waves with the parachute whilst people lie under it
- using a bubble blower and lava lamps.

A small, peaceful group session creates a space where people can make contact with each other – taking turns, passing instruments out, making gentle physical and social contact. The aims of these sessions focus on process rather than outcome. In a good session everyone:

- is heard
- listens to and makes contact with everyone else in the group
- leaves the room happy and relaxed.

Individual goals might include things like smiling, making eye contact, taking the opportunity to initiate a sound, a relaxation in posture or a reduction in biting or screaming. After the noise and energy of the larger group the absence of songs and even words can be quite intimidating. It's easy to miss or under-estimate what is achieved. Well-trained and supported support staff are essential to these sessions having value.

Exploring personal tastes

Sometimes people have had very limited access to different types of music and sometimes people get very stuck on one thing, maybe even one song. Small groups are a positive, gently sociable way of listening to things that either are new to everyone or that are shared by one person with the rest of the group. Human beings are often a bit sceptical about new things so it's useful to develop some approaches to respectfulness: when someone brings a CD by their favourite band no one else says they hate it and everyone tries, at least, to listen to it. It's possible (though maybe not always necessary or desirable) to link things in a way that makes them more likely to be listened to positively: Abba is often an easy step away from nursery rhymes, minimalism is a gentle introduction to classical music, classical music that is familiar to people because of adverts and films (see 'Enabling Participation in Music', Chapter 8) can be used as a step towards a broader listening to classical music.

Some of the people I work with have very specific hyper-sensitivity to particular frequencies or timbres of sound and in a large group with lots of things happening it can be hard to work out what those are. Small groups are a good forum for experimenting with different types of sound. The presence and support of others encourages people to try things. Caution is needed when exploring these kinds of sound preferences. It's important to try a little at a time and always to start quietly (see Working with people who have sensory disturbances, Chapter 7).

Small groups are a good place to introduce and experiment with playing new, and perhaps more challenging, instruments (accordion, harp, violin, sax, flute, clarinet, bass guitar). Many instruments are initially really difficult to get to sound and most instruments take quite a lot of co-ordination and dexterity. It's helpful for people to watch each other learning and trying but it takes time and focus; in a small group people don't lose interest waiting for their turn.

Teaching basic instrument skills

Teaching basic instrument skills sometimes works well in a small group. Learning to play an instrument well takes a lot of practice and a lot of effort. Some of the people in the group have only ever done things (music or otherwise) that someone else has decided will be easy for them to achieve; they may well not be used to a lack of immediate success. Keen guitar wannabes can soon be put off when it hurts their fingers, would-be rock drummers might well not anticipate how much clapping in time they are going to have to do to make it sound like anything other than a noise. Instrument teaching in a small group gives people chance to see that it's difficult and that the difficulty is not personal to them; it's difficult for anyone. It also makes it possible to produce results more quickly by splitting tasks between group members (e.g. taking one chord each).

Working on composition and performance

It's certainly possible, and great fun, to compose or perform songs (see 'Enabling Participation in Music', Chapter 8) as a large group activity but when it comes to fine tuning melody, harmony, instrumentation and/or lyrics a small group works better and gives the people involved a real opportunity to actively participate in the decisions that are made about the song. It's just not possible to do everything by large committee; it was no accident that the Beatles were 4 and not 12 and even then the song writing was, on the whole, 2 not 4.

Band rehearsals and ensemble practice are a rather different type of small group. When working on rehearsing a new song, putting together a performance or preparing for a recording we have rehearsals with a rehearsal schedule. This type of music group requires the commitment of its group members. People need to stick with the same instrument, learn their lyrics and so on. In these groups I do behave more directively, as I would with any group of musicians. I do also encourage much more critical appraisal (that was good – could it be better? How?). The people in the group are often more used to being told that everything they do is good or certainly having someone other than themselves be the judge of the quality of their performance. If they are serious about being taken seriously, in life, as well as in a band, they need the opportunity to develop the ability to accurately appraise, analyse and develop their own performance.

One-to-one sessions

One-to-one sessions are good for focusing on:

- specific instrument skills
- something an individual finds challenging or difficult
- individual composition.

Teaching specific instrument skills

Teaching techniques (right-hand playing styles for guitar, different drum kit patterns, two hand keyboard playing, saxophone embouchure, etc.) works best one-to-one, so that attention is focused entirely on the learner and teaching can be specifically tailored. Tailoring can take the form of very specific activity analysis and step-by-step building of skills (particularly when someone is very motivated to achieve something that's technically difficult), as it would in any one-to-one music lesson. These sessions need to be backed up with significant amounts of individual practice – learning to play an instrument is 99 per cent practice (see Craig's journey, Chapter 9).

Focusing on difficult or challenging musical ideas

Sometimes it's impossible for people to get the support they need with a specific task as part of the group (see Gavin's journey, Chapter 9).

Working on individual composition

Some of the songs the band has written are personal and are written in one-to-one sessions (see lyrics to Hi I'm Jamie in Appendix 1). I act as supporter and advisor and we make sure we get a finished, recorded result. It's a really productive way for people to show the world a little of who they are.

The large and small group sessions and one-to-one sessions are inter-connected. People use what they learn from one-to-one sessions to get more out of group time. People find out for themselves what they are capable of in a setting where it's easier to be heard, to concentrate, to find their place in the room and then take this back into the large group. As facilitator I take what

I learn about how people work, what they enjoy and what they bring and that informs how I facilitate the large group. When someone (an individual or a small group) has been working on something specific, perhaps a new song or a new instrument skill, the larger group is often the audience for our premier performance.

CHAPTER 13

Reflection

Coming up with ideas for sessions

The world is full of ideas but ideas can be rather like buses; sometimes they arrive in herds...sometimes they are entirely elusive. It's useful to have some strategies.

- Always carry a note book – things you see and hear, things that make you laugh, things you learn, stories you're told are all potential material.

- Don't ignore the everyday things – sometimes they're an inspiration!

- Often one idea will generate a whole set of others – make sure you write them down so they aren't lost.

- Whether it's the internet, the newspaper, a book or magazine – read looking for ideas, and you'll find some.

- Keep all your session plans and flick through them from time to time. Use them to trigger new ideas, or revisit and repeat things that it's useful to reinforce.

- Use what happens in one session to inform what you plan for the next.

- Sometimes less is definitely more. Plan some relaxed sessions and leave space for new things to emerge.

- Use models, theories, shapes and processes to re-focus, re-frame and re-think to stop things becoming stale.

- Generate activity ideas by drawing a page of music pies – put a music word in each – and fill them up with the other words that would make up the pie...

Music pies

- So first word is – jazz – the others could be – blues, bee bop, reggae, samba.

- Or they might be – standards, chord progressions, improvisation, modern, traditional, New Orleans.

- Or they might be – rock, pop, folk – whatever you like.

- First word is – volume – the others could be duration, movements, tempo.
- First word is   trumpet – the others could be tuba, trombone, French horn, cornet.
- Or they could be flute, clarinet, violin.
- For example, first word is…

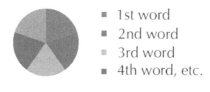

- 1st word
- 2nd word
- 3rd word
- 4th word, etc.

Figure 13.1 Music pies

Working out 'How?'

In the right circumstances people are capable of achieving incredible things.

- Think about how to break activities down.
- Believe that everything is possible. If an activity seems impossible it's because there's a different way of doing it that you haven't thought of yet.
- Look after yourself, if you can't give 100 per cent take a holiday.
- Don't under-estimate the value of repetition: gaining musical expertise, in whatever guise, takes huge amounts of practice.
- Have the time it takes to get there.
- Notice and remark upon the small gains along the way.
- Enjoy the journey.
- Appreciate and celebrate success magnificently.
- Always have fun.

Why music?

I never doubt that music adds value. Often what happens is amazing, moving, exciting, emotional and just being there to be part of it is incredible. For the people I work with music is so important and for me, like Frank Zappa (Sullivan 2003), it is the best.

I'm a fully paid up member of the blowing your own and everyone else's trumpet society. I'm incredibly proud of what we achieve, collectively and individually, and we celebrate in big and small ways as often as we can find an opportunity.

When I started this journey, five years ago, I thought I didn't need to be a registered OT any more. What I know now is I couldn't do what I do if I wasn't an OT; it is part of what makes it work.

We all 'do things' every day, that is 'human occupation'. The value in what I do is in its simplicity: to see the joy on someone's face when they clap in time, when they are heard, when they invent lyrics from imagination needs no scientific investigation or jargon – being the person who is there to see it is, quite simply, amazing.

It seems appropriate that my bit of this book does not end the book, but stops here by returning to Paul Abberley.

Paul felt that the problem with OTs was that their professionalism is founded on the dependency of disabled people (Abberley 1995). Applying a Social Model approach to OT practice is, I'm convinced, the way forward.

Acknowledgement

As part of the process of writing this book Jessica Kingsley Publishers offered to release some of The LA Buskers original songs and the Big Red Recording Studio, Dame Hannah at Seale-Hayne (www.discoverhannahs.org/Music/) generously donated their time, talents and recording studio to record them for us. We'd like to say a very big thank you to Jessica Kingsley Publishers and Dame Hannah's at Seal Hayne (and especially to Owen).

And so the book ends here with a few words from The LA Buskers about our time at the Big Red Recording Studio and their first experience of recording.

The LA Buskers

Before

How are you feeling about going to do the recordings?

Marie: We're going to have a good time, it'll be fun. I'll probably be nervous about going in the car. I've learnt all my words… I'll have to take my fags and Jane says I need to dress cool because we're filming.

Craig: I'm really excited; I've never seen a recording studio. I'm not nervous about anything – I love being in the band and I'm good at the bits I do in the songs.

Gavin: There are lots of things to think about because I've never been to a recording studio before. I might be a bit excited and a bit nervous. I'm looking forward to seeing Russell Watson again. I've seen him before, but next time I see him I'll tell him that I have recorded some tracks too.

Which song are you looking forward to doing most?

Marie: Tell Me What You Wanna Say – I like the way it sounds when we do it.

Craig: The Colgate Blues, it's funny.

Gavin: I'm looking forward to recording the tracks – including Scaletrix and Stickle Bricks and Pandora. Pandora is a song we did about meeting a girl for the first time and asking her to dance with me.

During

Marie: (Hearing our first track played back through the PA system.) That's me, that's me singing – I sound really good. Owen, thank you for letting us do this.

Gavin: It's interesting...

Cassie: I like it here. It's exciting...and it's so big, taller than Trago Mills.

After

Gavin: Are we going to the recording studios next week? When can we record all our other songs? Will people buy our CD in the shops? I did the bass line on Pandora. I'm pleased with the recordings and with the songs we did, I like Pandora best.

Marie: The recording studios were fantastic. I enjoyed being there with everyone. It was a fantastic day hearing my voice and the drums.

Cassie: The recording studio is very, very, very good. I played the xylophone with Annie and had hot drinks from the machine – it went beep but you didn't need to put any money in. I sang on Scaletrix and Stickle Bricks with Jane and Jamie – I wish I could fly – it's a lovely song. I want to play the recordings to my Mum; she will say it is very, very nice.

Jamie: Sounds good doesn't it? I've got a great voice, it's a good song.

You can download the recorded tracks from www.jkp.com/catalogue/book/9781849053068.

And the next step of the journey starts here... Everyone who dreams has music.

The lyrics to some of our songs

The first five are available to download as MP3 files from www.jkp.com/catalogue/book/9781849053068

Tell Me What You Wanna Say [#1 from www.jkp.com/catalogue/book/9781849053068]

Chorus
Tell me what you wanna say,
Tell me what you wanna say – tell me, tell me now coz I am listening.
Tell me what you wanna say,
Tell me what you wanna say – tell me, tell me now coz I am listening.

Verses
I don't care that much for toast and I don't like Tai Chi,
I would rather have a fag and another cup of tea…please.
I don't really much like rice but it's not as bad as a run,
Media studies with David is nice and music with Jane is usually fun.

I don't like bad messages on my Facebook page,
I would rather that people were nice.
One day I'd like to be on stage.
I don't much like coffee and I never drink tea.
Monday nights are happy ones coz then I can watch Glee.

I'd like you to listen to me sing, I want to go adventuring.
I would like to shop for stuff and I like trampolining.
I like writing songs with Tom and I like Ruby – yeah, yeah and yeah.
I like working on the farm and I quite liked Tony Blair.

Music makes me happy, there's songs I like to share,
Paul and me sing while we work. I hate that voice on 'Go Compare'.
I don't much like sad songs and I don't like 'Paint it Red',
I love to dance to 'Call on Me' and I like to stay in bed.

What it Would Be Like to Be [#2 from www.jkp.com/catalogue/book/9781849053068]

I have often wondered what it would be like to be
The very famous captain of the Yellow Submarine –
To float under the ocean whilst the band begins to play
And if the Beatles came to town I'd moor up in the Bay.

Or maybe I would rather be the driver of a bus
Take famous people shopping for their toys at Toys 'R' Us.
I'd pick up Lady Ga Ga, a pop star that I like,
She'd come to Toys 'R' Us and buy a sparkly silver bike.

What it would be like to be...
What it would be like to be.
What it would be like to be...
What it would be like to be.

Perhaps I'll build a space ship and travel off to Mars,
Take a trip with Major Tom and hang around the stars.
Just take a starring role: You be donkey, I'll be Shrek.
Do the swamp karaoke; get a glow like 'Ready Brek'.

Would Russell Watson join us? What song would he do?
If he sang 'Go Compare' we'd listen all the way through or...
I could just be Gavin, and I could be Marie
...maybe I'll be Craig then. Let's get Jane a cup of tea.
Now the sun is shining and this song is nearly done,
Let's stop and have some lunch, next week we'll write another one.

What it would be like to be (x3)
What it would be like to be – me.

Pandora [#3 from www.jkp.com/catalogue/book/9781849053068]

Out with my Mum, shopping for a new look,
Trying to be independent but she has the cheque book.

She's there, she's there, she's there – it's Pandora.
She's there, she's there, she's there...oh, if you saw her –
She's opened the lid, I can't get rid of the feelings I have for Pandora...

Tell her she's beautiful, ask if she likes my jeans...

Walking with my mates, on our way to the pub,
One of the gang, part of the club.
She's there, she's there, she's there – it's Pandora.
She's there, she's there, she's there…oh, if you saw her –
She's opened the lid, I can't get rid of the feelings I have for Pandora…

Tell her she's beautiful, ask if she'd like a drink…

At the disco, sipping a coke,
Trying to act cool – a real, cool bloke.
[*Do that chorus again, do that chorus again, DO THAT CHORUS AGAIN*]
She's there, she's there, she's there – it's Pandora.
She's there, she's there, she's there…oh, if you saw her –
She's opened the lid, I can't get rid of the feelings I have for Pandora…

Tell her she's beautiful, ask her to dance with me…

The Colgate Blues [#4 from www.jkp.com/catalogue/book/97818
49053068]

Woke up this morning,
Went to brush m' teeth
Picked up the toothbrush
Went to get the paste…someone'd pinched the Colgate
Got the Can't Find My Colgate Blues.

Woke up this morning,
Pulled up the shades.
Hoping for sunshine,
But the sky was grey… Think it's gonna rain,
Got the Bad Weather Blues.

Woke up this morning,
Went to have me fag.
Wind was blowing
Got my lighter out my bag… Couldn't get a flame
Got the Fag-Free Blues

Woke up this morning,
Switched on the TV.
Screen was flickering,
There was no picture for me…took it back to Argos
Got the No TV Blues.

Woke up this morning
Went to play my uke.

String was broken
Made me wanna puke… Can't tune my lele
Got the No Music Blues.

Hi I'm Jamie [#5 from www.jkp.com/catalogue/book/9781849053068]

1. I like to feel the rain on my face,
To be outside, have plenty of space.
I like to be quiet and listen to the sounds
Of outside happening all around.

Chorus:
Hi, I'm Jamie. How are you?
Did you have a good day? Has the sky been blue?
I like the grey days, the cold and the rain – even the ice won't make me complain.

2. Sometimes I sit under the tree,
Reading the paper, with a hot cup of tea.
I like to watch films on TV,
A chat with Mum and Dad is always nice for me.

Chorus

Instrumental Break

3. When I sit and have time to dream,
Of all the things that I have seen,
What I think is – I'm a lucky man,
I'm happy being who I am.

Chorus

It's Been a Good Day [not downloadable]

I played on the computer
We all went for a walk
And we had hot soup for our lunch
We had plenty of time to talk… It's been a good day.

Chorus: nah nah nah nah nah

Today we did some different things
And we all took turns to sing.
I worked outside where there's lots of room –
Space around me is a good thing… It's been a good day.

Chorus

We listen to music, choose what's for lunch
And here's our plan for the day
Plenty of hugs and plenty of laughs
Share the games we like to play… It's been a good day.

Chorus

Sometimes we paint, sometimes we draw
Or we might watch a DVD
But there always time to have a chat
And make a cup of tea… It's been a good day.

Instrumental

It's been a good day.

It's Good to Know what your Favourite Things Are [not downloadable]

Verse:
Gavin wants to fly to the States,
For his birthday – he thinks that will be great.
Take your shades Gav, cos you'll need to look cool.
Do you think that they show Skins there?

Darren loves music and noise,
He likes jumping and a laugh with the boys.
He's a drummer and a xylophone king
And I hear he quite likes tractors.

Chorus:
It's good to know what your favourite things are
Do you want to go watch the stock car?
Take a picnic of doughnuts and cold beer for Craig
Cos it's gonna be a 'hot day'!
It's good to know what your favourite things are,

How'd you feel in a really fast car?
Do you love eating cake?
Playing air guitar?
Or would you rather be in the pool?

Verse:
Shane wants to be Spider Man.
With his papers, Pete's a handbag fan,
He likes music – Abba's his favourite band
And there's nothing quite like a hug.

White dogs make Nicola smile:
Take a photo, watch TV for a while,
Have a bike ride down the lane to the pigs
And we love 'Can't Stand the Rain' now.

Chorus:
It's good to know what your favourite things are
Do you want to go watch the stock car?
Take a picnic of doughnuts and some nice cold beer
Cos it's gonna be a 'hot day'.
It's good to know what your favourite things are
How'd you feel in a really fast car?
Do you love eating cake?
Playing air guitar?
Or would you rather be in the pool?

Verse:
If you pogo, then Sam is the one
Stick a track on and we'll jump just for fun.
Share a good book and a fresh apple juice,
Don't forget that he loves trees too.
Stuart is a man of few words
When he's happy, he can sing like a bird,
Hold a photo for us all to see
Take a walk 'til it's time for tea.

Chorus:
It's good to know what your favourite things are
Do you want to go watch the stock car?
Take a picnic of doughnuts and some nice cold beer
Cos it's gonna be a 'hot day'.
It's good to know what your favourite things are

How'd you feel in a really fast car?
Do you love eating cake?
Playing air guitar?
Or would you rather be in the pool?

Verse:
Spanish sunshine is what Marie would head for
Pack your laptop and put on some shorts,
Get some cheap fags at the duty free
But you'd miss your 'nice cup of tea'.
So then, are you listening to me?
Tell me, what do you want to be?
Cos we know that you can make real your dreams
But you got to know this one thing:

Chorus:
It's good to know what your favourite things are
Do you want to go watch the stock car?
Take a picnic of doughnuts and some nice cold beer
Cos it's gonna be a 'hot day'.
It's good to know what your favourite things are
How'd you feel in a really fast car?
Do you love eating cake?
Playing air guitar?
Or would you rather be in the pool?

Onomatopoeia [not downloadable]

1. We're tired of all this rain now
And the way the ground turns to sludge
We're bored of having cold feet now
This cold front needs to budge

Chorus 1
Onomatopoeia
Onomatopoeia
Let's go to the beach

2. We're dusting down the Porsche now
And taking off the top
We're getting good vibrations
And we aint gonna stop

Chorus 2
Vroom Beep Beep
Vroom Beep Beep
Let's go to the beach

3. We're going on a boat trip
We're going to check out the babes
They won't know what we're doing
coz we're gonna wear our shades

Chorus 3
Yeah Baby
Yeah Baby
Let's go to the beach

4. Drinking sex on the beach
Lying in the sand
Later we'll light the Barbie
Later we'll be the band

Chorus 4
123 123 12
123 123 12
Let's go to the beach

Popples Rap [not downloadable]

Once there was a creature,
She lived under the sink.
[Don't press the self-destruct button]
Her name was…Popples – The closet rap star
[Don't, don't don't believe the hype]

Under the sink, hoping for a night out.
Trying out m'spits, get the drain pipes out.
I could be a rap star – if I get my shoes right…
Don't don't don't believe the hype.

Off to the night club,
Open mic, dub club.
Popples gonna rap hot – tonight at the rap spot.
Gotta have my tea first – pie and chips and bier wurst.
Fill right up or else I'll bite their feet first.

Eight days Popples been under this sink,
Practising my rap, cold tea to drink.
Tonight even Russell Watson won't top me –
'Could it be magic?' – No way to stop me.
Tonight'll be my night – don't don't don't believe the hype.

Scaletrix and Stickle Bricks [not downloadable]

1. Swinging high I'm at the park
Next shoot down the slide
Pretend I am a butterfly on a multi-coloured ride.

Chorus: Scaletrix and Stickle Bricks I wish that I could fly,
Scaletrix and Stickle Bricks, build Lego to the sky.

2. At the fair, I'm eating dogs
The hot ones that don't bark.
Gonna bump into a yellow car
Coz I don't know how to park.

Chorus: Scaletrix and Stickle Bricks I wish that I could fly,
Scaletrix and Stickle Bricks, build Lego to the sky.

3. Home today we're dressing up,
Not witches – that's too scary.
I'll be Jack and look for giants
And you can be a fairy.

Chorus: Scaletrix and Stickle Bricks I wish that I could fly,
Scaletrix and Stickle Bricks, build Lego to the sky.

4. It's dark outside, it's time for bed.
Teddy's coming too,
Snuggle up and read a book,
Spin dreams the whole night through.

An introduction to some useful music theory

Introduction

A basic understanding of music theory can demystify the tasks of finding the chords to harmonise a melody, working out the notes you need to play an instrumental break in the appropriate key, doing your own version of a popular song or writing an original one. Some basic concepts are outlined here: if you'd like to know more there's a plethora of music theory books, though some of them are a bit difficult to follow. Maureen Cox's *Music Theory: Grades 1–5 In a nutshell* (2012) is a good starting point, particularly for people who like to learn from pictures and diagrams rather than lots of words.

The music theory that underpins the music of the western world has a strong keyboard bias. If you're struggling to understand a concept it may help to try it out on a piano or keyboard. Playing piano keyboard gives visual clues and the relationship between natural pitches (white notes) and sharps and flats (black notes), the pattern of a scale and the shape of a basic chord are easier to follow if you can see as well as hear them.

Notes in music

Musical notes are named after the first seven letters of the alphabet: ABCDEFG. These are repeated along the length of the keyboard. Notice the way the black notes are grouped alternately in twos and threes. The white note to the immediate left of a group of two black notes is always C.

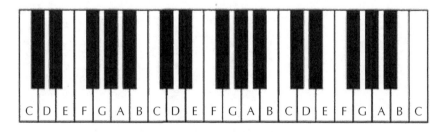

Figure Appx 2.1 Part of a piano keyboard

Each note can also be sharp (#), that is, a little higher in pitch, or flat (♭), a little lower in pitch. On a keyboard the sharps and flats are the black notes.

Sharpening an A gives A#, flattening a B gives B♭. A# and B♭ are the same pitch: the black note between A and B.

The distance between the notes on a keyboard (whether two white notes as in E to F or a white and a black note as in G to G#) is called a semi-tone (S). Two semi-tones (the distance between D and E for example) make a tone (T).

The distance between one C and the next (one B and the next, one D and the next, etc.) is called an octave (because it's eight notes).

A scale is a pattern of rising and/or falling notes. Western classical music tends to be based around three types of scale: major, minor and chromatic. If you're going to write songs the blues scale is useful too.

Major scale

The doe, ray, me, far, so, la, ti, doe in the song Doe a Deer is a major scale. Regardless of what note you start singing it on, the relationship between the notes of the scale is the same, that is, the scale has the same melody. (The words to Doe a Deer reflect the tonic sol-fa system used to teach music.)

The simplest major scale to play on a keyboard is C major. Start on C and play only the white notes: C D E F G A B C

In order to play this same melody starting on a different note you'd have to use some black notes too. Try G major: G A B C D E F# G or F Major: F G A Bb C D E F

If a melody starts and ends on C and only uses white notes then it is *in the key of C.*

If a melody starts and ends on G and uses an F# then it *is in the key of G.* (If you'd like to understand more about the relationship between keys look up The Circle of Fifths. The Circle of Fifths is a diagram that explains the tonal relationship between all the major and minor keys.)

The melody of the scale stays the same because the relationship between each note and its neighbours (whether they are separated by a tone (T) or a semi-tone (S) stays the same. The relationship between two notes (the number of semi-tones that separate them) is called an *interval.*

The intervals of a major scale are always: T, T, S, T, T, T, S

You can start a melody on any note. As long as you preserve the intervals between notes the melody stays the same.

With this knowledge you can:

- change the key of any melody to make it easier to sing

- change the key of any melody to a key you can play the chords for to make it instantly playable (see notes on harmony below)

- select a group of notes that work well together and use a random approach (see Developing skills in composition and song writing in Chapter 8) to compose a melody.

(Pop and folk music often stays in the same key, or very close to it, throughout. Classical music tends to change key as it unfolds…it's much easier to cover a pop song, knowing only three chords, than a symphony!)

Minor scale

Major scales are useful for writing bright, happy songs. If you want something sadder, moodier or a little more exotic try a minor scale. My favourite song written in a predominantly minor key is Killing Me Softly.

As with the major scale it's the intervals between the notes that matter – you can start on whatever note you like. The intervals of a minor scale are: T, S, T, T, S, T+S, S

The simplest minor scale is a minor: A B C D E F G# A – just one black note.

Blues scale

Again, with the blues scale, it's the intervals that are important: T+S, T, S, S, T+S, T.

So a C blues scale is: C E♭ F F# G B♭ C

…and usefully a blues scale has six notes, so it's an ideal candidate for composition by dice (see Chapter 8, 'Enabling Participation in Music').

Chromatic scale

A chromatic scale can start on any note and includes every note of the keyboard in order (i.e. every natural, sharp and flat). For example, the chromatic scale starting on C is C C# D D# E F F# G G# A B♭ B C

Harmony and basic chords

A chord is the sound you get when you play more than one note at a time. Chords come in all shapes and sizes, from simple to very complex; some are easy on the ear, some much harder to understand. For straightforward song writing and song performance all you need is an understanding of the simplest chords.

The most important chords to any key are the I, IV and V. In the key of C these are the chords of C, F and G (because in C C=I, D=II, E=III, F=IV, G=V, A=VI, B=VII).

In G they are G, C and D.

In D they are D, G and A. (D is a good key for guitar players: D, G and A are fairly easy chords to play and are often the first ones taught. If these are the only three chords you know just change the key of the melody of any song and play it in D.)

In its simplest form a chord comprises three notes: the note the chord is named after (C in the chord of C) then the next two alternate notes (for C – E and G). If you try it on a keyboard you'll see you are playing alternate notes.

Having chosen the key you are going to play in work out the three chords you need and try each one out against the melody: one of the three is bound to work (because one of the notes of the chord will be the same as the melody note…read some music theory if you'd like to learn more).

Setting up instruments to make instrumental breaks and/or chord playing accessible

Once you understand how to work out what key you're playing in then instruments can be set up to play only the notes of that key. This means that instrumental breaks and chord accompaniment can both be achieved successfully.

- **Some instruments are key specific** – For example a harmonica. If you don't know the key of your harmonica it's almost certainly C: Jam (make it up) over 12-bar blues in C (see Appendix 3) and you'll hear…it works. (Listen to Gavin play the harmonic break on The The Colgate Blues (www. jkp.com/catalogue/book/9781849053068).

- **Other instruments can be made key specific**

- **Keyboard** – Colour-code the notes using stickers (see colour-coding in Chapter 8).

- **Xylophone, glockenspiel, chime bars, handbells** – Remove the notes that aren't in the key you're playing in.

- **Guitar and ukulele** – Chords can be marked with colour-coded stickers or instruments can be open-tuned. (Open-tuning a stringed instrument means changing the pitch of the strings so that strumming the strings producing the notes of the chord without needing to hold strings down in a chord shape, e.g. to open-tune a ukulele to play in C the four strings, would be tuned to C, E, G and C.)

- **Tuning a string** – The note a string produces is made higher, in pitch, by tightening it and lower by loosening it. Use a digital tuner or Phone App to tune to the desired pitch.

Composition templates

A bar is a rhythmic building block. The time signature (the numbers at the beginning of a piece of music) state how many beats there are in a bar. Unless the time signature changes during the piece then each bar will have the same number of beats. Most pop songs are in 4/4 (four-four time): that means there are four beats in a bar. Dances (think about a waltz) are often written in 3/4 time: there are three beats in a bar. Marches are often in 2/4 – two beats in a bar (like walking as in the Pictures at an Exhibition Promenade, see Activity Plan 3).

Usually (there are many exceptions – reggae is perhaps the most obvious) the first beat of the bar is the most important and is therefore emphasised. In 4/4 the third beat is *usually* the next most important.

Composition blocks

A simple table can be used to represent a repetitive rhythm. I call it a composition block (Hanke 2003a). The composition block below illustrates a basic rhythm in 4/4. This same rhythm can be used with any pop song that's written in 4/4.

TABLE APPX 3.1 BASIC RHYTHM IN 4/4

Instrument	Beat: 1	2	3	4
Tambourine	X x	X x	X x	X x
Drum	X	X	X	X
Bell	x		x	
Bass drum	X			

Chord/phrase/cadence shape

Musical language has a lot in common with spoken language. Regardless of the form (whether a song or a symphony) the micro-level will be made up of phrases and these will have the musical equivalents of punctuation (capital letters, full stops, commas) in order to make sense.

Music, like poetry, is easiest to follow if the phrases are of equal length (four or eight bars is good).

Melodically, the strongest sense of capital letter (beginning) and full stop (end) is achieved by playing the tonic note (the note that names the key you're playing in, i.e. C if you're playing in the key of C).

Commas and full stops at the end of phrases are called cadences. The strongest sense of full stop (the end) is produced harmonically by playing the chords VI: this is called a perfect cadence. (Beethoven often repeats the perfect cadence several times, using it percussively, at the very end of a movement so that you are left in no doubt that it's the end.) In C the chords VI are GC.

One way of achieving a comma is to play an imperfect cadence by playing the chords IV (in C this is CG).

Imposing this structure by using a template will give a composition logical flow. A discernible beginning, middle and end will help to make it make musical sense. The template below gives a space to write the melody notes (that can be produced by the methods described in Chapter 8).

Start and end your melody on the tonic note, impose cadences at the end of regular phrases and you can produce a convincing tune at the throw of a dice.

TABLE APPX 3.2 MELODY TEMPLATE

Bar 1	2	3	4
			I V
5	6	7	8
			V I

Twelve-bar blues template

Twelve-bar blues is a prescribed harmonic rhythm (set of chord changes), much like the chord/phrase/cadence template above. Lots of very successful popular songs use 12-bar blues as a template – Elvis Presley's Jailhouse Rock, lots of Beautiful South's Don't Marry Her and Joan Lett's I Love Rock and Roll are all good examples.

The chord progression for 12-bar blues in C (or any other key) looks like this.

TABLE APPX 3.3 12-BAR BLUES CHORD PROGRESSION IN C

Bar	1	2	3	4	5	6	7	8	9	10	11	12
Chord	C	C	C	C	C	F	F	C	C	G	F	C
Chord No.	I	I	I	I	I	IV	IV	I	I	V	IV	I

Writing a song

Use the notes of the blues scale in your melody, and start and end on the tonic note.

Use the composition blocks to write your rhythm. Use either the 12-bar blues or cadence template to prescribe your chord pattern and you've got the music for a song – just add lyrics!

Once you've played with it a few times you'll want to try some different things – make it up, read some music theory or borrow some ideas from your favourite tracks. Enjoy!

APPENDIX 4

List of songs and instrumental works mentioned in the book

John Cage	4 minutes 33 seconds
Queen	We will Rock You
Beethoven	Symphony No. 5
Gerry Rafferty	Baker Street
Stravinsky	The Rites of Spring
Dvořák	New World Symphony
Bach	Air on a G string
John Williams	Theme from Jaws
Herrmann	Music from the *Psycho* shower scene
Strauss	Also Spracht Zarathustra (used for *2001: A Space Odyssey*)
Prokofiev	Peter and the Wolf
Shostakovich	Symphony No. 5
Elgar	Pomp and Circumstance March
Traditional	The ABC song
Beethoven	Violin Concerto
The Proclaimers	500 Miles
Paul Simon	50 Ways to Leave your Lover
Hancock	Chameleon
Procol Haram	A Whiter Shade of Pale
Greg Lake	I Believe in Father Christmas
Prokofiev	Sleigh Ride from Lieutenant Kijé
Mike Batt	Minuetto Allegretto (from The Wombles)
Mozart	Minuet from Jupiter symphony
Purcell	Dido's Lament (from Dido and Aeneas)
Tina Turner	Can't Stand the Rain

The Muppets	Mahna Mahna
Tchaikovsky	1812 Overture
Mendelssohn	Fingle's Cave
Vaughan Williams	London Symphony
Sant-Saëns	Carnival of the Animals
Mussorgsky	Pictures at an Exhibition
Don McLean	Vincent
Chopin	Nocturnes
Beethoven	Symphony 5
Vangelis	Mare Tranquillitatis
Holtz	Planet Suite
Britten	Sea Interludes
Queen	We will Rock You
Ravel	Bolero
Meatloaf	Bat out of Hell
Status Quo	Rocking all Over the World
Bob Marley	Buffalo Soldier
Adam and the Ants	Prince Charming
Traditional	Ten Green Bottles
Traditional	Old MacDonald
Traditional	How Much is that Doggy?
Traditional	The Runaway Train
Baha Men	Who Let the Dogs Out?
Traditional	Went to the Animal Fair
Lulu	Shout
Traditional	The Lambeth Walk
Traditional	What Shall We Do with a Drunken Sailor
Traditional	She'll be Coming Round the Mountain
Louis Armstrong	Wonderful World
Cat Stevens	Morning has Broken
John Lennon	Imagine
Grease	You're the One that I Want
Grease	Born to Hand Jive
Maceo Parker	Rabbits in the Pea Patch
Jamiroquai	Feel so Good

Traditional	The Okey Cokey
Traditional	Head and Shoulders
Traditional	One Finger, one Thumb
Traditional	If You're Happy and You Know It
Ritchie Valens	La Bamba
Los Del Rio	The Macarena
The Gap Band	Oops Upside Your Head
Richard O'Brien	The Time Warp
Bobby Picket	The Monster Mash
Brenda Lee	Jump the Broomstick
Traditional	The Wheels on the Bus
Joan Jett	I Love Rock 'n' Roll
Westbrook	Trifle
Ella Fitzgerald	One Note Samba
John Lennon	Lucy in the Sky with Diamonds
The Village People	YMCA
Peter Gabriel	Kiss that Frog
Lou Reid	Perfect Day
Nizlopi	JCB Song
Ian Dury	Spasticus Autisticus
Ian Dury	Profoundly in Love with Pandora
Snow Patrol	Chasing Cars
Pärt	Spiegal im Spiegal
Grease	Sandra Dee
Traditional	Ging Gang Gooley
Traditional	Thank You Very Much
The Troggs	Love is all Around
Bruno Mars	Just the Way You Are
Roberta Flack	Killing Me Softly
Einaudi	Due Tramonti
Nyman	The Heart asks Pleasure First (theme from *The Piano*)
Chubby Checker	The Twist
The Contours	Do You Love Me (Now That I can Dance)
Elvis Presley	Jailhouse Rock

Chuck Berry	Johnny be Good
The Police	Walking on the Moon
Barry Gray	The Thunderbirds March
David Bowie	Space Oddity
Bach	Cello Suites
Vangelis	Mare Tranquillitatis
Music Express 5	Spacescape
Maroon 5	She Will be Loved
REM	Bad Day
Strauss	Till Eulenspiegel
Sibelius	5th Symphony
Tchaikovsky	Swan Lake
Tchaikovsky	The Nut Cracker Suite
Prokofiev	Romeo and Juliet
Rorem	Picnic on the Marne
Maurice	Tableaux de Provence
Bruno Mars	The Lazy Song
Mussorgsky	Night on a Bare Mountain
Traditional	Campfire's Burning
Traditional	You'll Never go to Heaven
Traditional	Do Your Ears Hang Low?
Manfred Mann	Do Wah Diddy Diddy
Tommy James and The Shondells	Mony, Mony
Elton John	Crocodile Rock
Joni Mitchell	Big Yellow Taxi
Katrina and the Waves	Walking on Sunshine
The Blues Brothers	Minnie the Moocher
Arthur Hamilton	Sing a Rainbow
Chris de Burgh	Lady in Red
UB40	Red, Red Wine
Nena	99 Red Balloons
Howard Goodall	Theme from Red Dwarf
Traditional	Oranges and Lemons
REM	Orange Crush

Lennon and McCartney	Yellow Submarine
Dawn	Tie a Yellow Ribbon
Coldplay	Yellow
Shakin' Stevens	Green Door
Rodgers and Hart	Blue Moon
Prince	Purple Rain
Britten	Night Mail
Gershwin	Rhapsody in Blue
Cliff Richard	Summer Holiday
The Beach Boys	Good Vibrations
Fidler's Dram	Day Trip to Bangor

Inventory of instruments, equipment and resources

Here's a list of the instruments and equipment mentioned in the book. Most of the things on the list aren't costly and some can be picked up at your local scrap store or recycling centre.

Instruments:

- Drum sticks
- Cajon (sit on wooden drumming boxes)
- Toms and djembes
- A drum kit
- A drum machine
- Tuned percussion: chime bars, xylophone, glockenspiel
- Untuned percussion: tambourines, guiros, castanets, shakers, wood-blocks, wobble-boards, cabasas
- Boom whackers
- Coloured handbells
- Ukuleles
- Guitar slides
- Cymbala
- Squeeze box/harmonium/accordion
- Harmonicas
- Piano keyboard.

Equipment:

- Multi-coloured parachute
- Mirrors (a range of hand mirrors and large wall mirrors)
- Large foam dice, soft balls, balloons, skittles

- Coloured cloth, scarves and ribbons
- Pom-poms (cheerleader-style)
- Exercise balls or space hoppers
- A hammock or swing
- Wrist and ankle weights
- Mechanical microphones
- Cordless microphones
- An amplifier
- Voice changers
- A conducting baton
- Puppets
- Story Cubes (The Creativity Hub)
- Art and craft materials.

Resources:
- Digital tuner
- Metronome
- Digital recorder
- Multi-media projector
- Camera
- Camcorder
- Laptop
- Digital desk toys that react to sound
- Audacity (music editing free-ware available at http://audacity.sourceforge. net, accessed 7 February 2013)
- eJay (composing software).

References

Abberley, P. (1995) 'Disabling ideology in health and welfare – The case of Occupational Therapy.' *Disability and Society 10*, 2, 221–232.

Abbott, J. and Marriott, J. (2012) 'Money, finance and the personalisation agenda for people with learning disabilities in the UK: some emerging issues.' *British Journal of Learning Disabilities 40*, 1. Advance online publication.

Adams, D. (1995) *The Hitch-hiker's Guide to the Galaxy: A Trilogy in Five Parts*, 1st edn. London: William Heinemann.

Amnesty Magazine (2011) 'Esa-Pekka Salonen.' Issue 70, Nov/Dec 2011, 38.

Ayres, J. (1979) *Sensory Integration and the Child*. Torrance, CA: Western Psychological Services.

Barenboim, D. (2008) *Everything is Connected: The Power of Music*. London: Weidenfeld and Nicolson.

Barnes, C. and Mercer, M. (1996) *Exploring the Divide: Illness and Disability*. Leeds: The Disability Press.

Berne, E. (1985) *Games People Play: The Psychology of Human Relationships*. London: Penguin Books.

Brammer, A. (2010) *Social Work Law*, 3rd edn. Harlow: Pearson Education.

Brewer, M. (2002) *Mike Brewer's Warm Ups!* Harlow: Faber Music.

Bonetti, R. (2006) *Confident Musical Performance: Fix the Fear of Facing an Audience*, 2nd edn. Sydney: Taking-Centre Stage.

Caldwell, P. (2008) *Using Intensive Interaction and Sensory Integration. A Handbook for Those who Support People with Severe Autistic Spectrum Disorder*. London: Jessica Kingsley Publishers.

Campbell, D. (1997) *The Mozart Effect: Tapping the Power of Music to Heal the Body, Strengthen the Mind and Unlock the Creative Spirit*. London: Hodder.

Campbell, J. and Oliver, M. (1996) *Disability Politics*. London: Routledge.

Clements, L. (2012) 'Disability, dignity and the cri de coeur.' *European Human Rights Law Review* 6, 675–685.

Clements, L. and Read, J. (2008) *Disabled People and the Right to Life*. London: Routledge.

Cooke, D. (1959) *The Language of Music*. Oxford University Press. Re-issued in paperback, 1989: Clarendon Paperbacks.

Cox, M. (2001) *Music Theory: Grades 1–5 in a Nutshell*. Subject Publications.

Culham, A. and Nind, M. (2003) 'Deconstructing normalisation: Clearing the way for inclusion.' *Journal for Intellectual and Developmental Disability 28*, 1, 65–78.

Dahl, R. (1991) *The BFG; Matilda; George's Marvellous Medicine*. London: Jonathan Cape.

DeGraffenreid, G., Fowler, C., Gerber, T. and Lawrence, V. (2006) *Music! Its Role and Importance in our Lives.* New York, NY: Glencoe.

Doney, M. (2006) *Musical Instruments.* London: Watts Books.

DRC (2006) *Equal Treatment: Closing the Gap.* Part 1 of the DRC's Formal Investigation Report. Stratford upon Avon: Disability Rights Commission.

Duncan, E.A.S. (2011) *Foundations for Practice in Occupational Therapy.* London: Churchill Livingstone/Elsevier.

Equality and Human Rights Commission (2009) *An Effective Approach to Disability Discrimination in the Equality Bill.* London: EHRC.

Finkelstein, V. (1999) 'The Social Model of Disability and the Disability Movement.' In: E. Stone (ed.) *Disability and Development: Learning Form Action and Research on Disability in the Majority World.* Leeds: The Disability Press.

Goddard-Blythe, S. (2012) *The Genius of Natural Childhood: Secrets of Thriving Children.* Portland, OR: Hawthorn House.

Hagedorn, R. (1992) *Occupational Therapy: Foundations for Practice. Models, Frames of Reference and Core Skills.* London: Churchill Livingstone.

Hanke, M. (2003a) *Music Express 5 A and C.* London: Black.

Hanke, M. (2003b) *Music Express 6 A and C.* London: Black.

Hopkins, H.L. and Smith, H.D. (eds) (1993) *Willard and Spackman's Occupational Therapy,* 8th edn. Philadelphia, PA: JB Lippincott.

HSE (2003) *Health and Safety Regulation... A Short Guide HSE 13* (rev 1), revised 08/03. London: Health and Safety Executive.

HSE (2004) *Manual Handling. Manual Handling Operations Regulations 1992* (as amended). HSE books. London: Health and Safety Executive.

Hunt, P. (1966) 'A Critical Condition.' In T. Shakespeare (ed.) *The Disability Reader* (1998) London: Cassell.

Kielhofner, G. (1985) *A Model of Human Occupation: Theory and Application.* Williams and Wilkins: Baltimore, MD.

Kolb, D.A. (1984) *Experiential Learning: Experience as the Source of Learning and Development.* Englewood Cliffs, NJ: Prentice Hall.

Latham, A. (ed.) (2004) *Oxford Dictionary of Musical Terms.* Oxford: Oxford University Press.

Law, M., Baptiste, S., McColl, M. *et al.* (1990) The Canadian Occupational Performance Measure: An outcome measure for occupational therapy. *Canadian Journal of Occupational Therapy 57,* 2, 82–87.

Levitin, D. (2006) *This is Your Brain on Music: Understanding A Human Obsession.* London: Atlantic Books.

Mäkinen, K. (2009) *The Kalevala: Tales of Magic and Adventure.* Vancouver, BC: Simply Read Books.

Marsh, S. (2011) '*DDA RIP! What Next? Rights and Disabled People.*' Paper presented at The Centre for Disability Studies Seminar Series, University of Leeds, Leeds, 30 March.

Mattingly, C. and Flemming, M.H. (1994) *Clinical Reasoning: Forms of Inquiry in a Therapeutic Practice.* Philadelphia: FA Davis.

McCormack, C. and Collins, B. (2010) 'Can disability studies contribute to client-centred occupational therapy practice?' *British Journal of Occupational Therapy 73*, 7, 339–342.

Mithen, S. (2007) *The Singing Neanderthals: The Origins of Music, Language, Mind and Body.* Massachusetts: Harvard University Press.

Oliver, M. (1990) *Politics of Disablement.* Basingstoke: Macmillan.

Oliver, M. (1992) 'Changing the social relations of research production.' *Disability, Handicap and Society 7*, 2, 101–114.

Oliver, M. (2004) 'The Social Model in Action: If I Had a Hammer.' In C. Barnes and G. Mercer (eds) *Implementing the Social Model of Disability: Theory and Research.* Leeds: The Disability Press.

Oliver, M. (2009) *Understanding Disability: From Theory to Practice,* 2nd edn. London: Palgrave Macmillan.

Pallier, C., Christophe, A. and Mehler, J. (1997) 'Language specific listening.' *Trends in Cognitive Sciences 1*, 4, 129–132.

Patel, A.D. and Daniele, J.R. (2003) 'An empirical comparison of rhythm in language and music.' *Cognition 87*, 1.

Rink, J. (ed.) (2006) *Musical Performance: A Guide to Understanding.* Cambridge: Cambridge University Press.

Roberts, R. (2004) *Mood Music* [set of CDs]. Camarthan: Crown House Publishing.

Roth, I. (2010) *The Autism Spectrum in the 21st Century: Exploring Psychology, Biology and Practice.* London: Jessica Kingsley Publishers.

Sacks, O. (2008) *Musicophilia: Tales of Music and the Brain.* London: Picador.

Schon, D. (1983) *The Reflective Practitioner.* New York, NY: Basic.

Seuss Dr (1960) *One Fish, Two Fish, Red Fish, Blue Fish.* Beginner Books. New York: Random House.

Sullivan, P (2003) *Sullivan's Music Trivia.* London: Arcane.

Swain, J., Finkelstein, V., French, S. and Oliver, M. J. (eds) (1993) *Disabling Barriers – Enabling Environments.* Milton Keynes: The Open University and Sage Publications.

The Open University (2002a) *AA314 Studies in Music 1750–2000: Interpretation and Analysis.* Block 5 English Musical Identity c.1880–1939. Milton Keynes: The Open University Press.

The Open University (2002b) *AA314 Studies in Music 1750–2000: Interpretation and Analysis.* Offprints 2. Milton Keynes: The Open University Press.

Thomas, C. (2004) 'How is disability understood? An examination of sociological approaches.' *Disability and Society 19*, 6 22–36.

Thompson, R. (2011) *Musical Instruments.* London: Franklin Watts.

Tovey, D.S. (1944) *Beethoven.* London: Oxford University Press.

Williamon, A. (2006) *Musical Excellence: Strategies and Techniques to Enhance Performance.* Oxford: Oxford University Press.

Zarb, G. (2004) 'Independent Living and the Road to Inclusion.' In C. Barnes and G. Mercer (eds) *Disability Policy and Practice: Applying the Social Model.* Leeds: The Disability Press.

Further Reading

Craddock, J. (1996) 'Responses of the occupational therapy profession to the perspective of the disability movement – Part 1 and Part 2.' *British Journal of Occupational Therapy 59*, 17–22 and 73–78.

DoH (2010) *Prioritising Need in the Context of Putting People First: A Whole System Approach to Eligibility for Social Care.* Guidance on Eligibility Criteria for Adult Social Care. London: DoH.

French, S. (1994) 'Disabled People and Professional Practice.' In *On Equal Terms: Working With Disabled People.* Oxford: Butterworth-Heinemann.

Haddon, M. (2004) *The Curious Incident of the Dog in the Night-Time.* London: Vintage.

Hammel, K.W. (2007) 'Reflections on a disability methodology for the client-centred practise of occupational therapy research.' *Canadian Journal of Occupational Therapy 74*, 5.

Jongbloed, L. and Crichton, A. (1990) 'A new definition of disability: Implications for rehabilitation practice and social policy.' *Canadian Journal of Occupational Therapy 57*, 1, 32–38.

Kielhofner, G. (2005) 'Rethinking disability and what to do about it: disability studies and its implications for occupational therapy.' *American Journal of Occupational Therapy 59*, 5, 487–496.

The Makaton Charity (1996) *Makaton Core Vocabulary – Signs.* Pocket Books 1 and 2. Surrey: The Makaton Charity.

Mosey, A.C. (1981) *Occupational Therapy Configuration of a Profession.* Raven Press: New York.

Mosey, A.C. (1986) *Psychosocial Components of Occupational Therapy.* New York: Raven.

Mullins, L.J. (1999) *Management and Organisational Behaviour,* 5th edn. Upper Saddle River, NJ: Financial Times, Prentice Hall.

'Music Matters: Has Music Changed the World?' BBC Radio 3 Free Thinking Festival discussion programme broadcast live on November 5th 2011.

Oliver, M. (1996) 'Defining Impairment and Disability: Issues at Stake.' In C. Barnes and G. Mercer (eds) *Exploring the Divide: Illness and Disability.* Leeds: The Disability Press.

Pavlicevic, M. (1999) *Music Therapy: Intimate Notes.* London: Jessica Kingsley.

Ramey, M. (2011) *Group Music Activities for Adults with Intellectual and Developmental Disabilities.* London: Jessica Kingsley.

Schwarz, R. (2007) *Wind Chimes and Whirligigs (Kids Can Do It).* Toronto, ON: Kids Can Press.

Storms, G. (1998) *Handbook of Music Games.* London: Souvenir Press.

Storms, J. (1995) *Music Games for Children.* Alameda, CA: Hunter House.

Swain, P. and French, S. (2000) 'Towards an affirmation model of disability.' *Disability and Society 15*, 4, 569–582.

Web References

Audacity freeware. Available at: http://audacity.sourceforge.net/about, accessed on 28 November 2012.

Bailey, R. (2012) NHS: barriers to equal treatment. *Disability Now*. Available at: www.disabilitynow.org.uk/blog.nhs-barriers-equal-treatment, accessed on 28 November 2012.

Disabled People's Action network DAN (2012) Available at: www.disabilitynow.org.uk/article/meet-future-young-campaigners-show, accessed on 28 November 2012.

Effect of Music on Serotonin Levels. Available at: www.buzzle.com/articles/how-does-music-affect-the-brain.html, accessed on 28 November 2012.

Finkelstein, V. (2001) A Personal Journey into Disability Politics. Leeds University Centre for Disability Studies. Available at: www.leeds.ac.uk/disability-studies/archiveuk/finkelstein/presentn.pdf, accessed on 28 November 2012.

Heavy Load's home page. Available at: www.heavyload.org, accessed on 28 November 2012.

HMSO (1967) Abortion Act. Available at: www.legislation.gov.uk/ukpga/1967/87/pdfs/ukpga_19670087_en.pdf, accessed on 28 November 2012.

HMSO (1995) Disability Discrimination Act. Available at: www.legislation.gov.uk/ukpga/1995/50/section/1, accessed on 28 November 2012.

Mencap (2012) Death by Indifference. Available at: www.mencap.org.uk/campaigns/take-action/death-indifference, accessed on 28 November 2012.

MOHO resources including interest checklist. Available at: www.moho.uic.edu/mohorelatedrsrcs.html, accessed on 28 November 2012.

Occupational Therapy: Its Values and Beliefs. (COT 2004). Available at: www.cot.co.uk/ot-helps-your-client/definition-occupational-therapy-its-values-and-beliefs, accessed on 28 November 2012.

Poverty UK (2010) Long-term Working Age Recipients of Out-of-Work Benefits. Available at: www.poverty.org.uk/14/index.shtml, accessed on 28 November 2012.

Savill, R. (2003) *Telegraph* Newspaper. Available at: www.telegraph.co.uk/news/uknews/1447096/Curate-takes-police-to-court-over-abortion-of-cleft-palate-foetus.html#, accessed on 28 November 2012.

Slorach, R. (2011) 'Marxism and disability.' *International Socialism 129*, 4. Available at www.isj.org.uk/?id=7.2, acccessed on 6 February 2031.

Stay Up Late. Available at: http://stayuplate.org/about, accessed on 28 November 2012.

Social Model of Disability site for people who have been labelled as people with learning difficulties. Available at: www.peoplefirstltd.com, accessed on 28 November 2012.

The KAWA Model. Available at: http://individual.utoronto.ca/michaeliwama, accessed on 28 November 2012.

The Mozart Effect. Available at: http://lrs.ed.uiuc.edu/students/lerch1/edpsy/mozart_effect.html, accessed on 28 November 2012.

Web Further Interest

Accelerated learning methods. Available at: www.acceleratedlearningmethods.com/auditory-stimulation.html, accessed on 28 November 2012.

Classic FM's music charity. Available at: www.makingmusic.org.uk, accessed on 28 November 2012.

compuTR web design offers a range of free leisure interest checklists in different formats to download. Available at: www.computr.net/download2.htm, accessed on 28 November 2012.

Critical Incident Analysis. Available at: www.usabilitynet.org/tools/criticalincidents.htm, accessed on 28 November 2012.

Critical Incident Analysis. Available at: http://en.wikipedia.org/wiki/Critical_Incident_Technique, accessed on 28 November 2012.

Social Model of Disability. Available at: http://en.wikipedia.org/wiki/Social_model_of_disability, accessed on 28 November 2012.

Index